Patient Pictures

HIV medicine

by

Duncan Churchill MRCP

Lecturer and Honorary Senior Registrar

Imperial College School of Medicine at St Mary's,

Imperial College of Science, Technology and Medicine, London, UK

and

Valerie Kitchen FRCP

Senior Lecturer and Honorary Consultant

Imperial College School of Medicine at St Mary's,

Imperial College of Science, Technology and Medicine, London, UK

Series Editor

J Richard Smith MD MRCOG

Senior Lecturer and Honorary Consultant Gynaecologist

Charing Cross and Westminster Medical School,

Chelsea and Westminster Hospital, London, UK and

Honorary Consultant Gynaecologist

Royal Brompton Hospital, London, UK

Illustrated by

Dee McLean, MeDee Art, London, UK

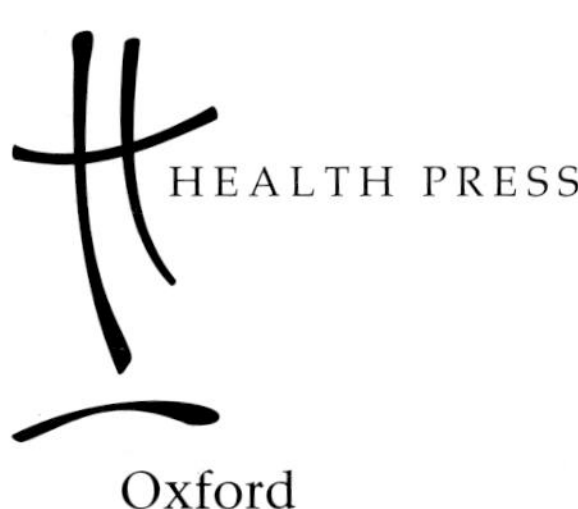

Oxford

Patient Pictures – HIV medicine
First published 1997

Elizabeth House, Queen Street, Abingdon, Oxford OX14 3JR

A CIP catalogue record for this title is available from the British Library.

ISBN 1-899541-90-X

Typeset by Impressions Design & DTP, Bicester, UK
Printed by Uniskill, Witney, UK

Contents

Reproduction authorization

Authors' preface

Acquired Immune Deficiency Syndrome or AIDS was first recognized in the early 1980s, and a blood test for the human immunodeficiency virus – HIV for short – became generally available in 1985. Since that time, our understanding of HIV infection and the medical conditions that arise as a result of the immune failure in AIDS, has become clearer. Preventive therapy for common infections and, more recently, combination drug therapy against HIV have been shown to have a dramatic impact on the quality of life and survival of infected patients.

Patient Pictures – HIV medicine explains the basic mechanisms involved in HIV infection, and the way in which anti-HIV treatments work. It offers practical advice for the prevention of HIV transmission, and deals with those questions most frequently asked in HIV out-patient clinics. This book has been designed to help healthcare professionals discuss the medical and surgical procedures that may be required during the investigation and treatment of HIV-related disease, with their patients. Although useful in its entirety, the sections do, as far as possible, stand alone.

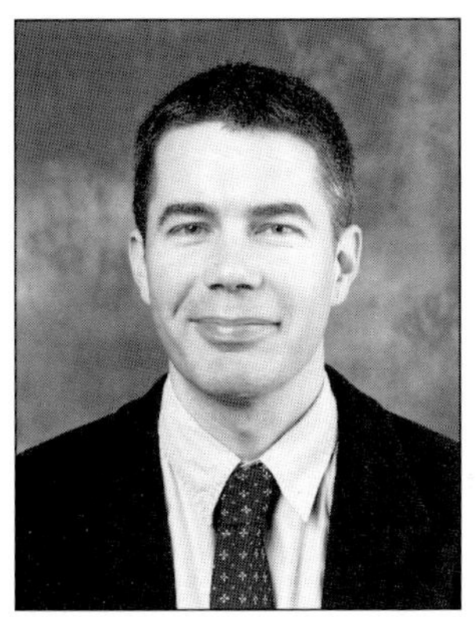

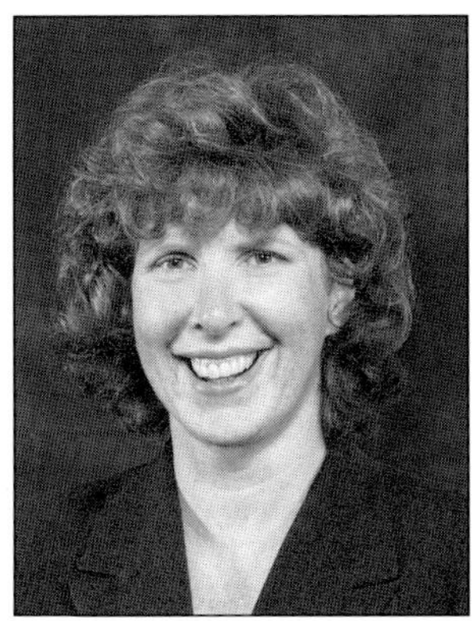

Duncan Churchill and Valerie Kitchen
Imperial College School of Medicine at St Mary's, London, UK

HIV transmission

- At the end of 1996, 22.6 million people in the world were thought to be infected with HIV.
- Like all human viruses, the human immunodeficiency virus or HIV, can only reproduce by infecting susceptible cells in the body.
- HIV is transmitted by the transfer of body fluids, particularly blood, semen and vaginal fluids, from an infected person to an uninfected person. This can occur through sexual contact, by sharing needles or by transfusion of infected blood. The virus can also be passed from mother to baby in the womb, and by breast-feeding after birth.
- HIV is **not** spread by touching, kissing or any other form of social contact.
- Whether or not you are infected, always use a condom for vaginal or anal sex. Try to limit your number of sexual partners.
- Always get prompt treatment if you think you have a sexually transmitted disease as some can make it easier for HIV to be passed on.
- Always use clean needles and syringes for injecting drugs and don't share needles.
- If you are HIV-positive, talk to your doctor about taking anti-HIV drugs during pregnancy, and ways to reduce the risk of passing HIV to your baby during labour. Don't breast-feed your baby.

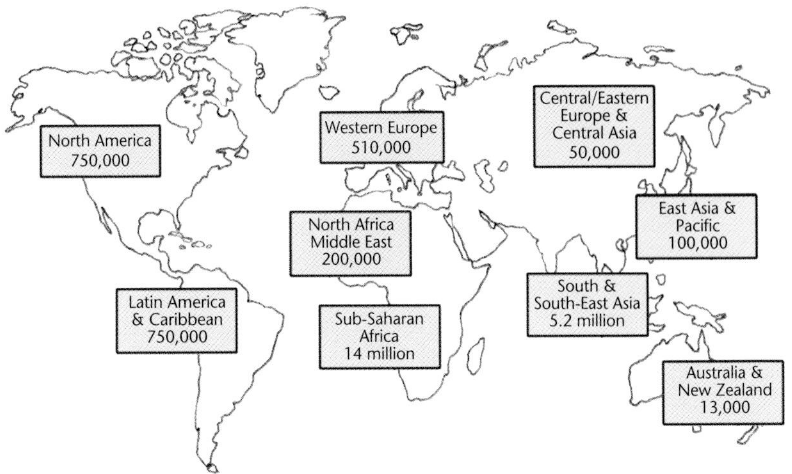

The estimated number of people living with HIV infection or AIDS at the end of 1996

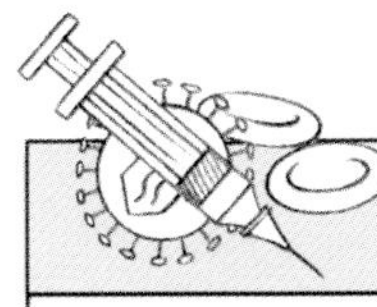

HIV INFECTION CAN OCCUR:

- during unprotected sex with an infected person
- by sharing needles and injecting equipment
- from blood transfusions with infected blood
- during pregnancy, from an infected mother to her baby
- during breast-feeding by an infected mother

Testing for HIV infection

- Your doctor will discuss the tests to detect HIV infection with you before they are carried out. Don't be afraid to ask questions if you don't understand.

- The tests involve looking for antibodies to HIV in a sample of blood. Antibodies are the body's infection-fighters, and are made when infection occurs. Different antibodies are made for different infections, and the antibodies made when HIV infects can be recognized by a laboratory test.

- The test is extremely sensitive, which means that it can detect very small amounts of antibody. If the HIV-specific antibodies are found in your blood, your test result is positive. If this happens, the sample is tested again using a different method to confirm the result. Your doctor will only tell you that you are HIV-positive if both tests are definitely positive.

- HIV tests will not give a positive result immediately after infection. It usually takes 2–6 weeks for the antibodies to become detectable in the blood, though it may take up to 3 months. This process of antibody production is called seroconversion. Until seroconversion has occurred, an infected person will give a negative test result as the antibodies are not in the blood and so can't be detected. If you have a negative result, you may be offered another test in 3 months' time.

- During the seroconversion time, the amount of HIV in the blood may be very high. This increases the chance that the virus can be passed on to an uninfected person, so it is important to follow your doctor's advice about reducing the risk of passing on HIV during this time.

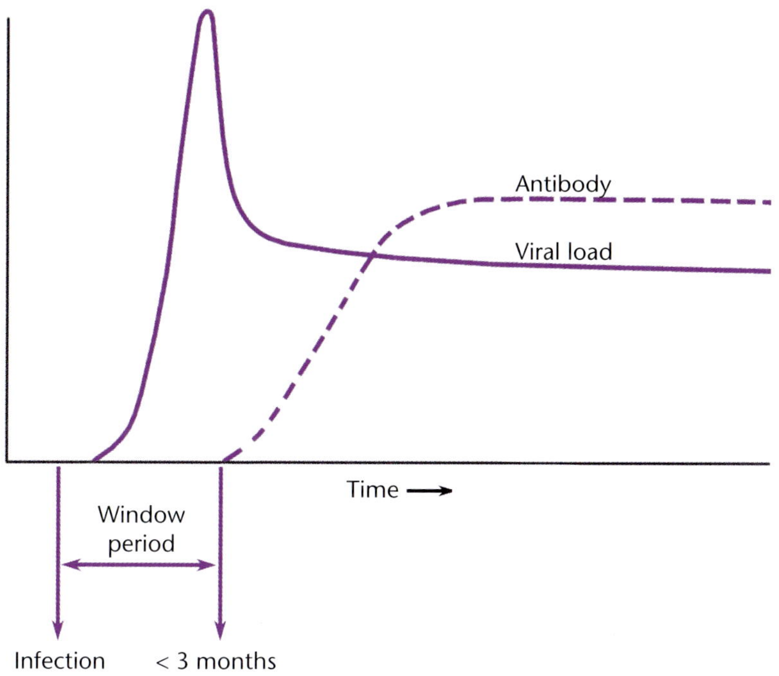

During the window period, the antibody to HIV cannot be detected, and an HIV test will give a negative result, even though the viral load is high

Seroconversion illness

- Around half of all people infected with HIV become recognizably ill at the time when antibodies to HIV appear in the blood. As this process is called seroconversion, the illness that occurs during this time is called seroconversion illness.

- Seroconversion illness usually happens 2–4 weeks after the person became infected, but may occur as early as 6 days or as late as 6 weeks after infection. It usually lasts for 1–2 weeks.

- The most common symptoms of seroconversion illness are fever, headache, skin rash, sore throat, enlarged lymph glands, nausea, vomiting and diarrhoea, and they occur as the virus spreads to susceptible cells in the body. It is important to remember that other viruses can also cause these symptoms.

- Occasionally, ulcers develop in the mouth, genital area or oesophagus.

- During seroconversion illness, patients may be more susceptible to other infections, such as thrush and, very occasionally, a particular form of pneumonia called *Pneumocystis carinii* pneumonia or PCP for short.

- After this time, people's resistance to infection usually returns to normal for several years until their condition worsens.

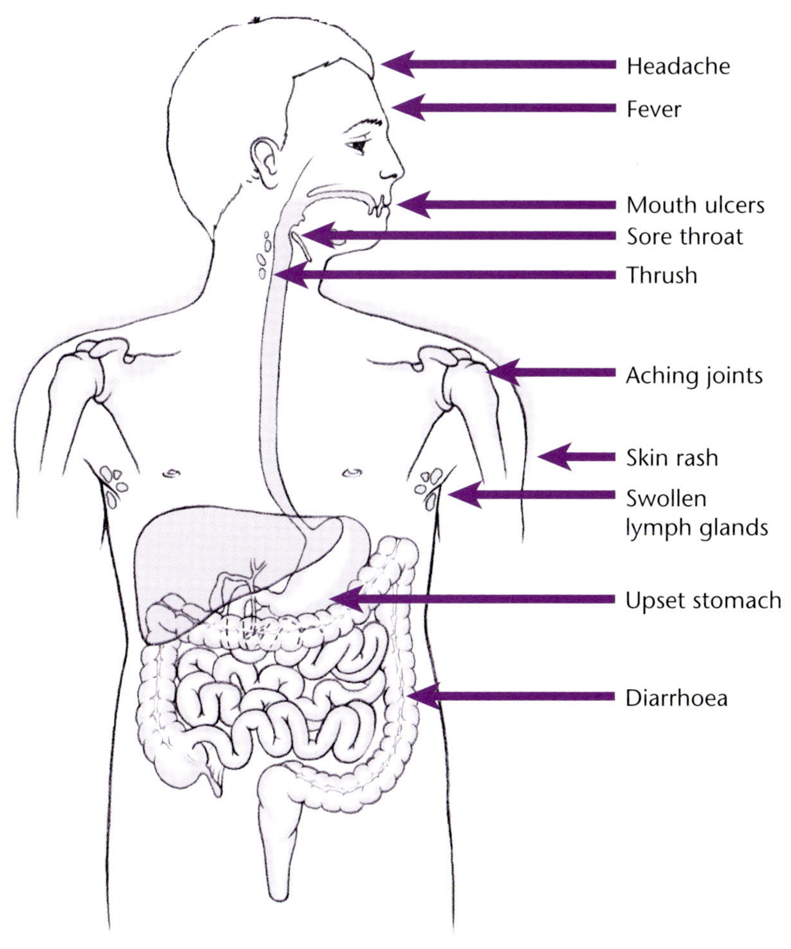
Headache
Fever
Mouth ulcers
Sore throat
Thrush
Aching joints
Skin rash
Swollen
lymph glands
Upset stomach
Diarrhoea

How AIDS develops

- Around half of people infected with HIV will develop AIDS after 10–11 years. Some people will remain well for considerably longer, while AIDS will occur more quickly in others.

- AIDS occurs when the person's immune system begins to break down. The immune system protects the body against infection and when it does not respond properly to infection, the person is said to be immunodeficient.

- As more effective and powerful drugs become available, it is likely that the average time between HIV infection and the development of AIDS will take much longer.

- Patients with AIDS become susceptible to a range of diseases that would not normally affect them if their immune systems were intact.

- Tumours, which are growths, may also occur. Common tumours that affect people with AIDS include Kaposi's sarcoma and certain kinds of lymphoma. Kaposi's sarcoma is a tumour that occurs in the skin and appears as a purple or dark brown patch. A lymphoma is a tumour that grows in the lymph gland.

- Following HIV infection, persistent enlargement of the lymph glands is common. Early signs that the disease is worsening include thrush in the mouth, unexplained fevers, night sweats, diarrhoea, weight loss and shingles.

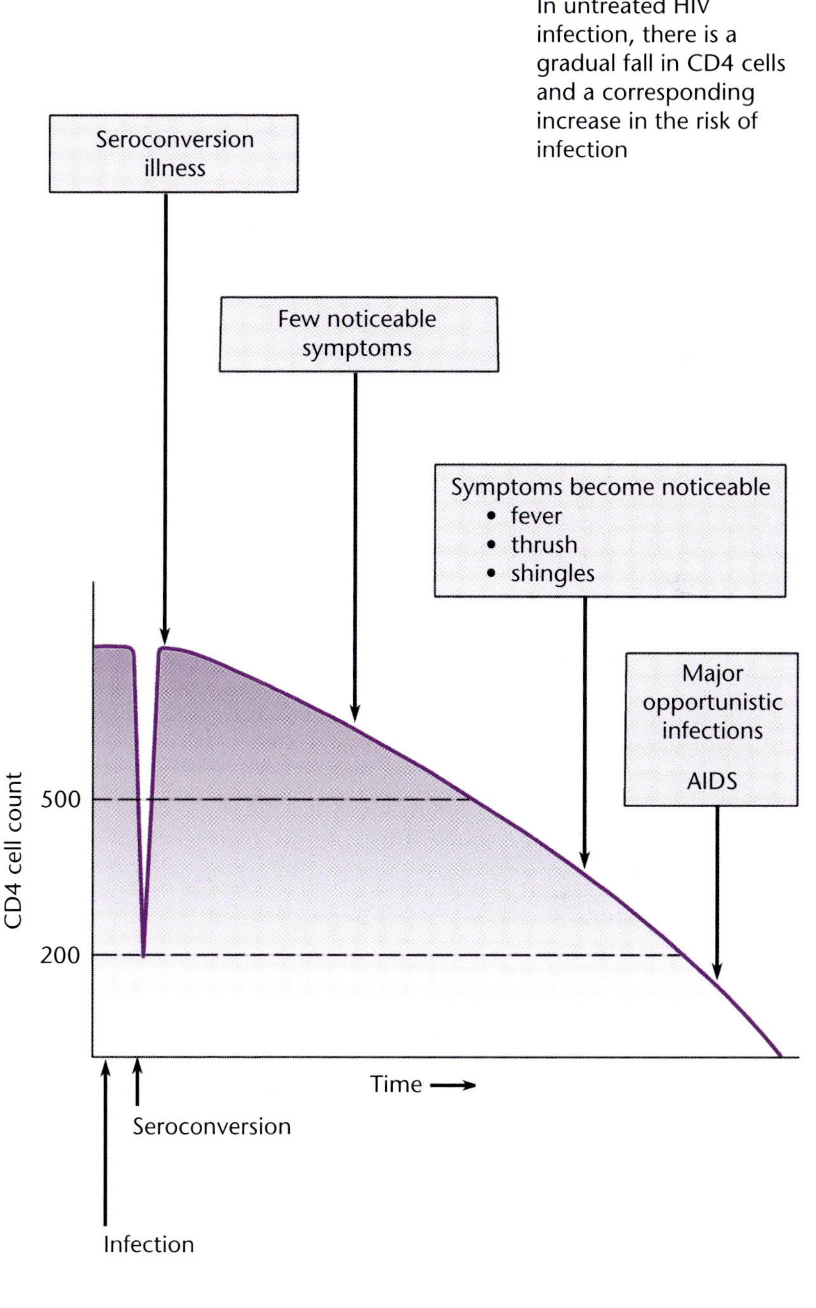

In untreated HIV infection, there is a gradual fall in CD4 cells and a corresponding increase in the risk of infection

Viral life cycle

- When HIV enters the body, it attaches itself to the surface of certain white blood cells in the blood. The most important of these are called CD4 cells, $CD4^+$ lymphocytes or T_4 cells.

- Once attached, the virus enters the cell and begins to make copies of itself. This copying process is called viral replication.

- The first step in viral replication depends on the action of a viral enzyme called reverse transcriptase. Enzymes are an important and complicated group of proteins that act to speed up events in the body that might otherwise be so slow that they never occur. Most currently available anti-HIV drugs work by blocking the action of reverse transcriptase so that the virus finds it difficult to make copies of itself. These drugs are called reverse transcriptase inhibitors.

- Another enzyme, called a protease, is needed by the virus to make more viruses that are able to infect new cells. Drugs have now been developed that block the action of this enzyme and these are called protease inhibitors.

- Mistakes called mutations often occur during the production of new viruses. These can lead to some drugs losing their ability to block the virus's enzymes. The virus is then said to be resistant to that particular drug. Treatment with combinations of drugs reduces the chance of drug resistance developing, so that the drugs can be used for a longer time.

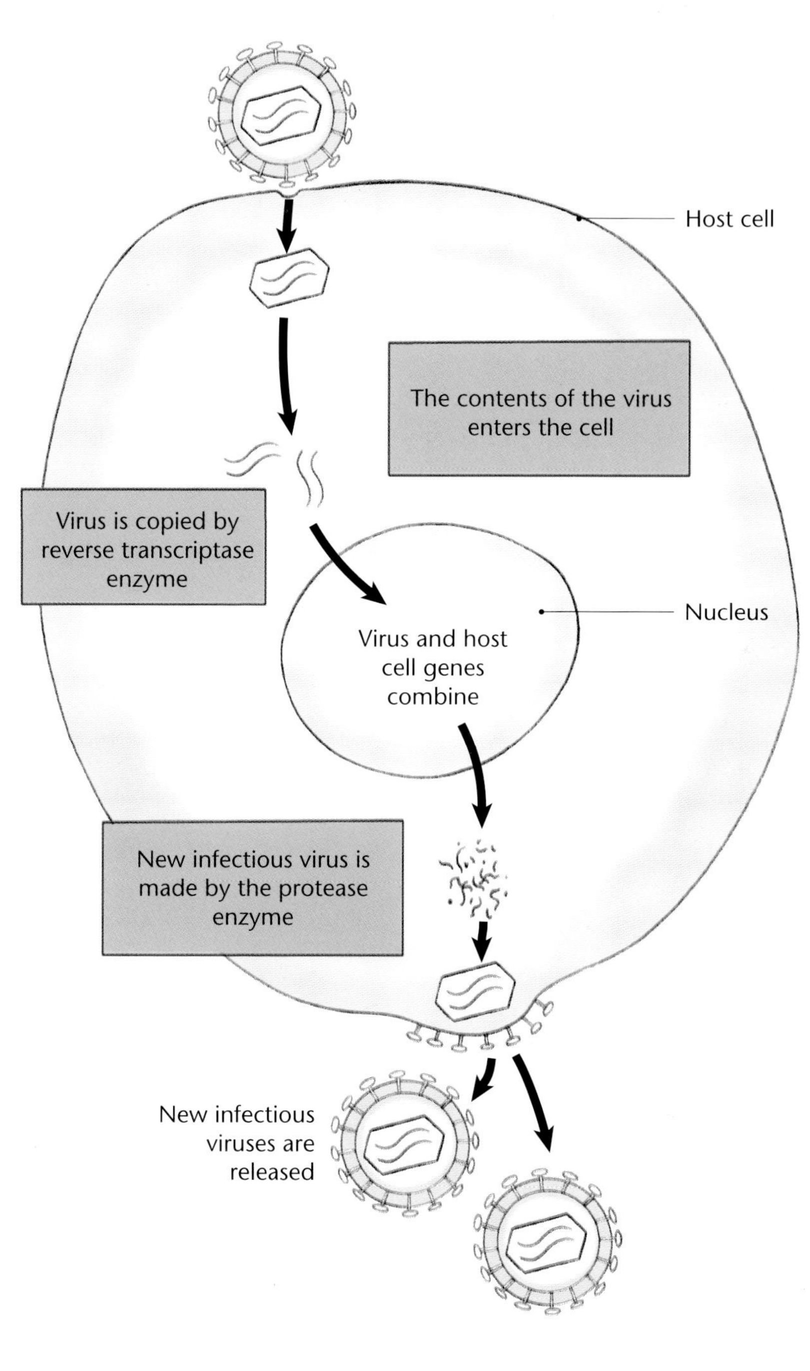
Host cell
The contents of the virus
enters the cell
Virus is copied by
reverse transcriptase
enzyme
Nucleus
Virus and host
cell genes
combine
New infectious virus is
made by the protease
enzyme
New infectious
viruses are
released

Anti-HIV drugs

- Drugs to treat HIV infection block the enzymes that the virus uses to make copies of itself.
- Drugs that work by blocking reverse transcriptase include zidovudine, which is often called AZT or ZDV.
- Drugs that block the protease enzyme include saquinavir, ritonavir and indinavir.
- Different drugs may cause different side-effects. Headaches, for example, are commonly experienced for a short time when starting AZT treatment.
- It is important to know about the side-effects that may occur with your drugs so that you can take steps to minimize them.
- As drugs have to be taken in different ways, take special care to read the dosing instructions. For example, saquinavir and ritonavir must be taken with food, while indinavir and didanosine must be taken on an empty stomach.
- Some drugs, particularly those that block the protease enzyme, interact with drugs used to treat other conditions. It is **very** important to tell your doctor about all the drugs that you take, whether they are prescribed or bought from a pharmacy. Some recreational drugs may also cause dangerous interactions with protease inhibitors.

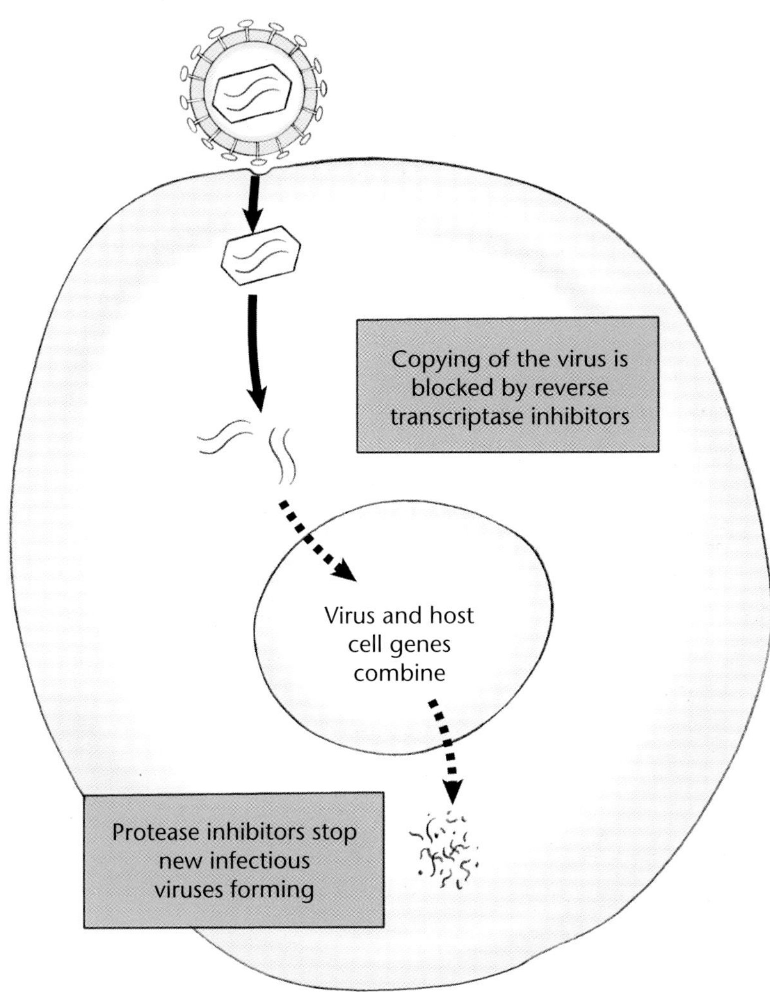
Copying of the virus is blocked by reverse transcriptase inhibitors
Virus and host cell genes combine
Protease inhibitors stop new infectious viruses forming

Monitoring drug treatment

- The effect of drug treatment is monitored by measuring the number of CD4 cells in the blood. They are the cells that are most susceptible to HIV infection and destruction. The amount of virus in the blood is also measured, and this is called the viral load.
- The number of CD4 cells and the viral load are usually measured before you start or change treatment, and then again 4–8 weeks afterwards.
- If your treatment is working, the number of CD4 cells in your blood will usually go up while the viral load will usually go down. If your illness is at an advanced stage, you may notice that your symptoms improve and you might put weight on.
- If the treatment isn't working, other drugs may be added to your treatment or you might be switched to different drugs.
- If the treatment is working, your CD4 cells and viral load will be measured every 3–6 months to check that the drugs are still working as time goes on. You might need different drugs if your viral load gets higher, your CD4 cell count drops, or if you develop new symptoms.
- It is important that you take your drugs correctly, and that you do not miss doses. Taking drugs incorrectly may give the virus a chance to make more copies of itself and so increase your viral load. It also may let the virus become resistant to a drug or drugs which will limit which drugs your doctor can prescribe for you in the future.

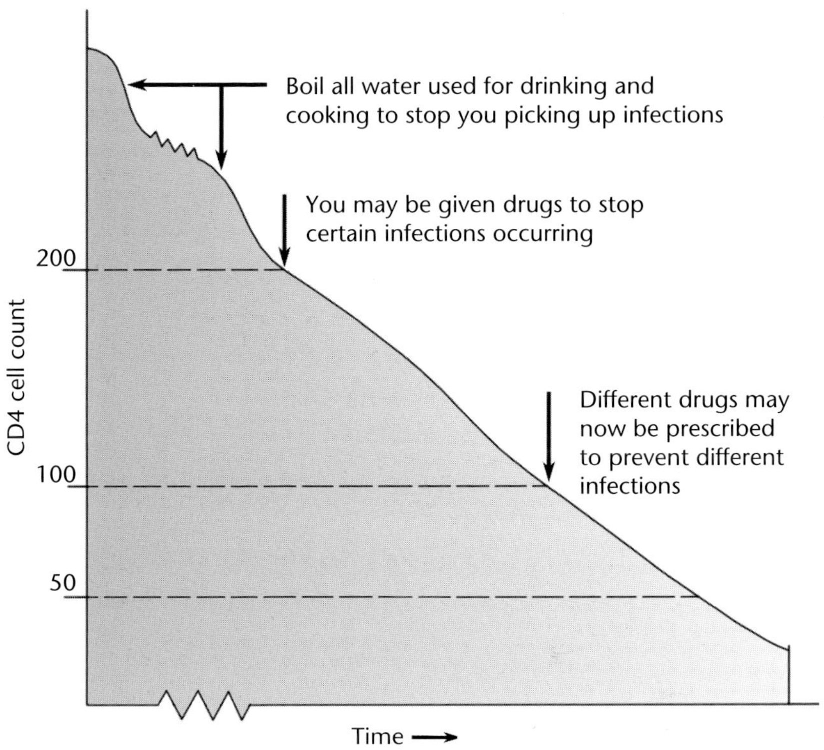

As your CD4 count drops, your doctor will advise you how to prevent infections, and prescribe certain drugs

Markers of disease progression

- Different blood tests can be used to assess the progression of HIV disease. Usually your CD4 cells and your viral load are measured. CD4 cells are the cells that are most susceptible to HIV infection and destruction. Viral load is the amount of virus present in your blood. These tests are normally performed every 3–6 months.

- Your number of CD4 cells, sometimes called a CD4 count, shows how well your immune system is coping. Using these measurements, your doctor can get an idea of your health over the next 6 months or so. CD4 counts can be affected by different things, such as illness, and so a single CD4 count can be misleading.

- Viral load measurements give your doctor an idea of how your disease would affect you in the longer term, if you did not have treatment.

- Your viral load may go up for a few weeks after a vaccination or if you have another infection, such as flu. Be sure to tell your doctor about either of these as your tests should be put on hold for a few weeks.

- Without treatment, some infected people have a viral load so low that it is not detectable using the usual methods. Some drug combinations can also reduce the viral load to this level, meaning that there are fewer viruses in the body and disease progression should be slower. Such low measurements **do not** mean that you are no longer infected.

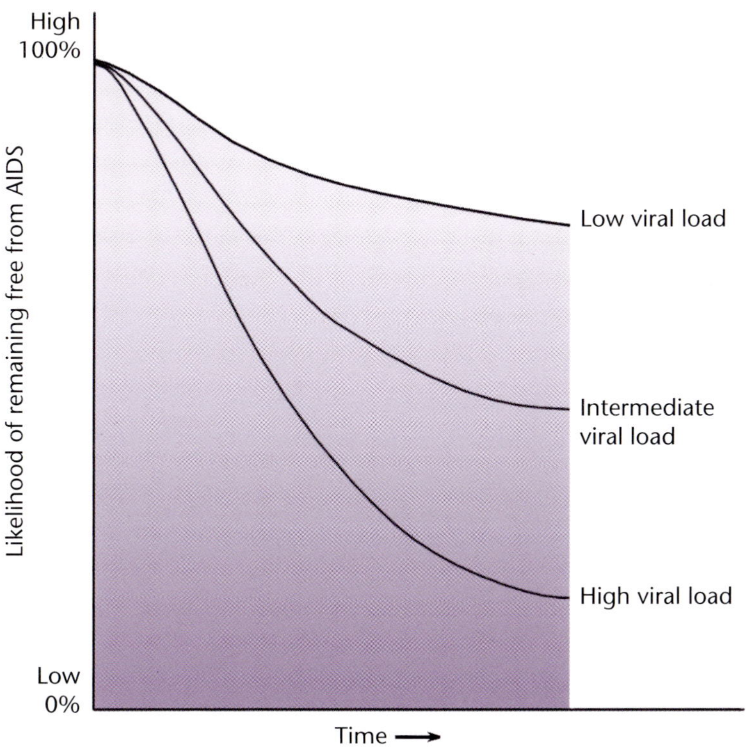

Your viral load measurement can be used to estimate how soon AIDS will develop

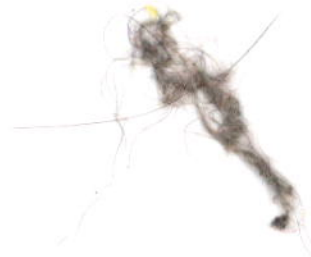

HIV and STDs

- Some STDs, short for sexually transmitted diseases, cause open sores or breaks in the skin in the vulva, vagina, rectum or on the penis. HIV can pass into and out of the body through these sores, so an STD puts an uninfected person at greater risk of becoming infected, and increases the chance of an infected person passing HIV on to their sexual partner.

- Condoms provide good protection against infection with HIV and other STDs.

- Infections such as genital herpes, vaginal thrush and genital warts are likely to become more severe and/or occur more often as the immune system begins to weaken and AIDS develops. When this happens, a longer or higher-dose treatment for these conditions may be needed.

- Pelvic inflammatory disease occurs when STDs affect the Fallopian tubes. As it may be more severe in people with HIV infection, bed rest and an injection of antibiotics may be needed.

- As STDs are often present without causing symptoms, many people do not know that they are infected. Because of the link between STDs and the spread of HIV, it is sensible to have regular check-ups for STDs.

FEMALE GENITAL TRACT

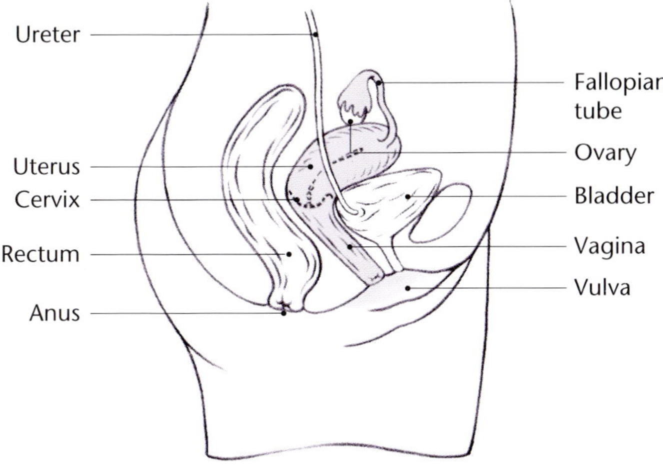

MALE GENITAL TRACT

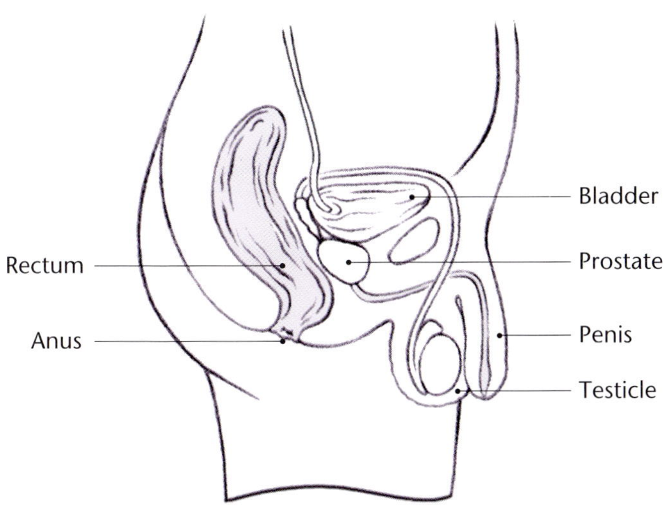

Pregnancy and HIV

- The risk of a mother transmitting HIV to her baby during pregnancy goes up if she has a low CD4 cell count or a high amount of virus in her blood. CD4 cells are the cells that are most susceptible to HIV infection and destruction.

- Although some babies are infected relatively early in pregnancy, most are infected around the time of delivery. Some babies are infected after birth as a result of breast-feeding by infected mothers.

- AZT, which is also called zidovudine or ZDV, may be prescribed any time after the 14th week of pregnancy. Normally, this drug is started between the 24th and 28th week. If you have been taking this drug already, you may be prescribed another drug called 3TC as well. AZT may also be given to your baby for the first 6 weeks of life.

- A long labour may increase the chance of passing HIV on to your baby so you may be advised to have a Caesarean section. This avoids the baby coming into contact with the HIV that is in the body fluids in your birth canal.

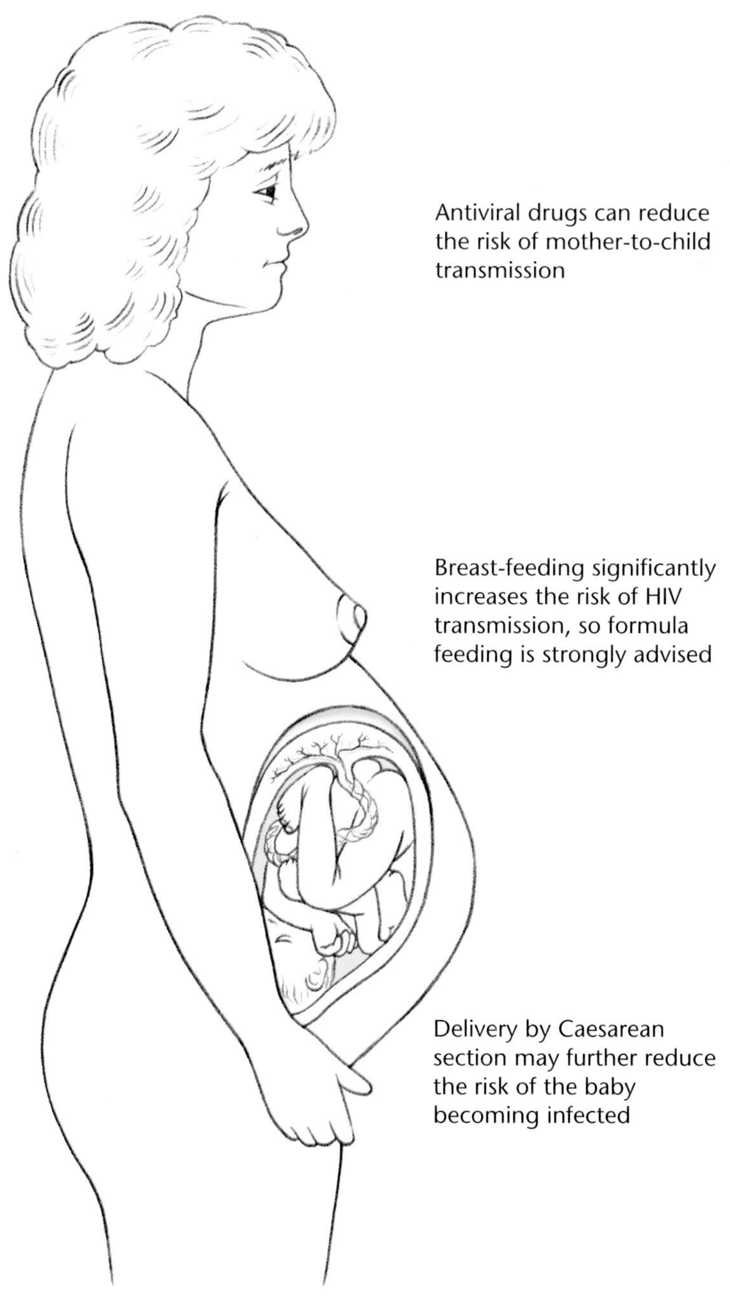
Antiviral drugs can reduce the risk of mother-to-child transmission
Breast-feeding significantly increases the risk of HIV transmission, so formula feeding is strongly advised
Delivery by Caesarean section may further reduce the risk of the baby becoming infected

Cervical cancer and colposcopy

- HIV infection itself does not lead to the development of cervical cancer. However, the effect of HIV on the immune system increases the risk of cervical cancer developing.
- If you are a woman with HIV infection, you are recommended to have a cervical smear test every 6 months or every year, so that any changes in your cervix can be detected early and treated.
- If an abnormality is detected on your smear, your cervix will be looked at more closely. This procedure is called colposcopy, and allows the doctor to get a magnified and clear view of your cervix. It is an uncomfortable but painless procedure and is carried out in the out-patient department. Colposcopy might also be done routinely every 6 months or every year if you are HIV positive.
- During colposcopy, dilute acetic acid and iodine may be painted onto the cervix in order to highlight any abnormal changes. This is also completely painless.
- A small piece of tissue may be removed and sent to the laboratory to be analysed. This sample of tissue, or biopsy as it may also be called, provides extra information about the cells in your cervix.
- You may bleed slightly after your biopsy has been taken but this is nothing to worry about.
- If an abnormality is seen during colposcopy, it can be treated under local anaesthetic.

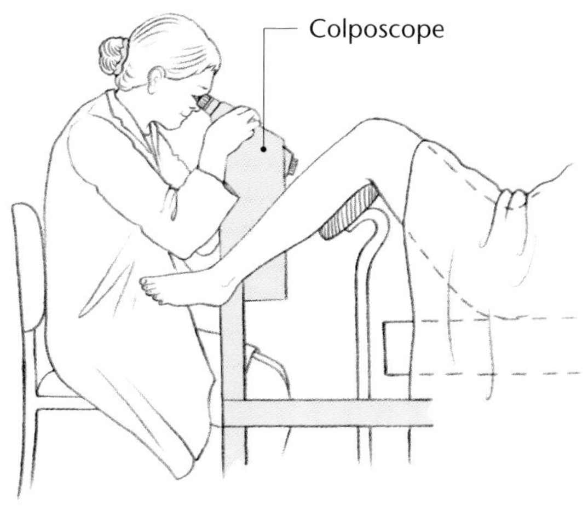
Colposcope

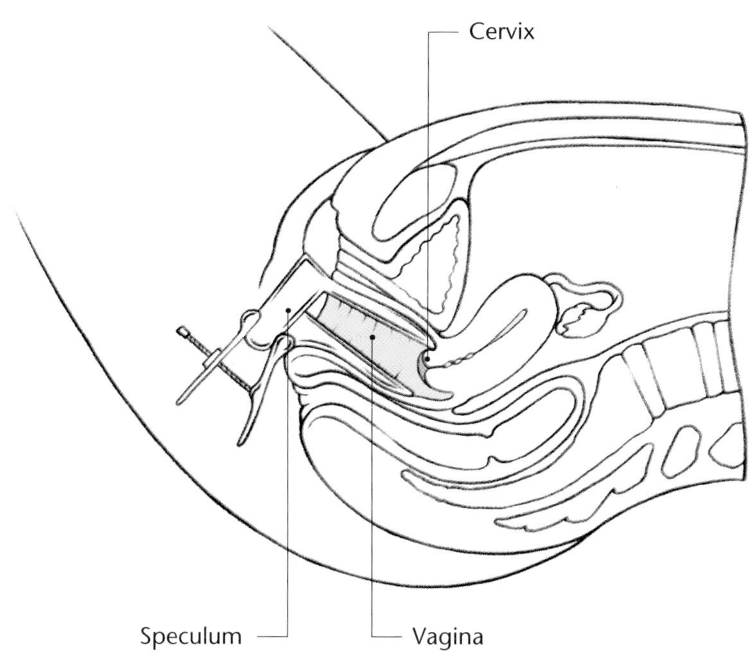
Cervix
Speculum
Vagina

Respiratory infections

- Infections that affect the lungs are known as respiratory infections. They are common in people with HIV infection, especially in smokers.

- Two infections that are particularly common are *Pneumocystis carinii* pneumonia which can be shortened to PCP, and tuberculosis or TB.

- Respiratory infections can be diagnosed using chest X-rays, a technique called bronchoscopy, or by examining sputum, which is the mucus or phlegm that is produced in your lungs if they are infected.

- A special technique called sputum induction is needed to diagnose PCP, as the infection is usually deep in the lungs. PCP cannot normally be diagnosed by ordinary sputum examination.

- For sputum induction, you will be asked to breathe in a fine mist of a salty solution, which is produced by a machine called a nebulizer. When the salty mist is inhaled deep into your lungs, it will make you cough up some sputum. This will be collected and examined in the laboratory. No anaesthetic or sedative drugs are needed for sputum induction.

- Sometimes, in order to make a diagnosis, your lungs will be examined using a fibre-optic 'telescope' called a bronchoscope. This way of examining your lungs is called bronchoscopy.

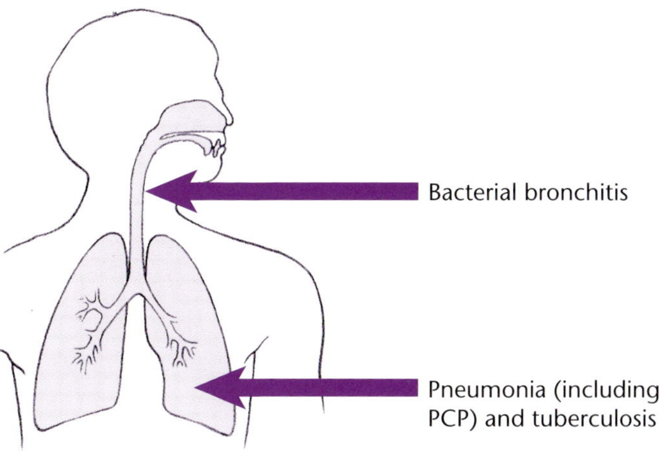

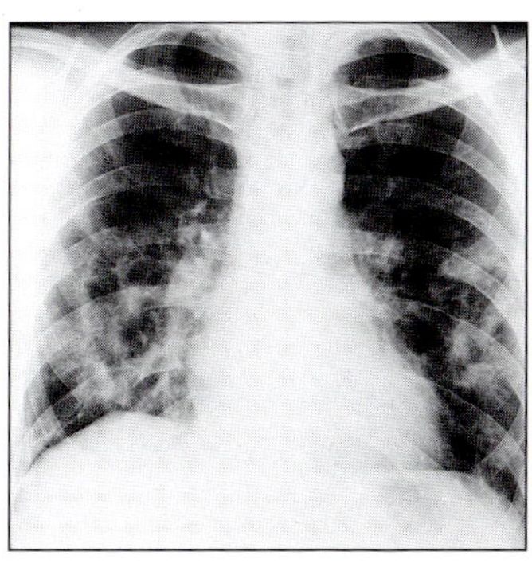

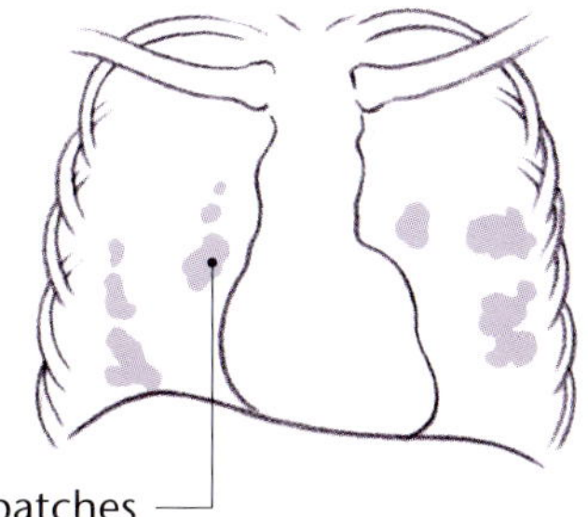

X-ray shows typical changes with pneumonia

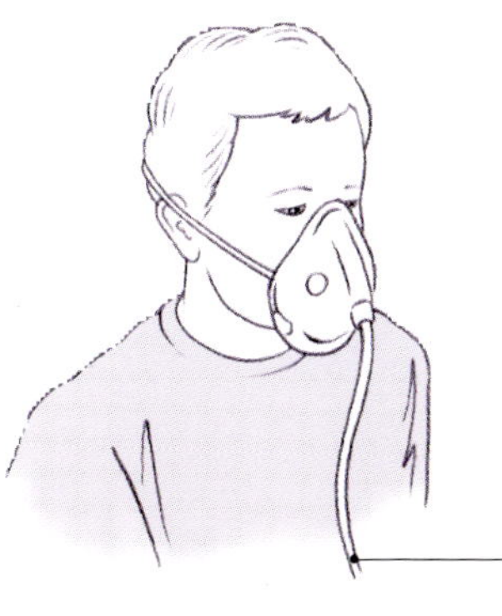

Bronchoscopy

- With bronchoscopy, the lungs are examined using a flexible fibre-optic 'telescope' called a bronchoscope.
- Bronchoscopy is usually performed as an out-patient procedure and takes about 1 hour. You must not eat or drink from the night before the examination.
- Local anaesthetic will be sprayed into your nose and mouth to make you more comfortable and stop you coughing during the procedure. A sedative and an injection to dry up the secretions in your lungs and windpipe may also be given.
- The bronchoscope is inserted through the nose and is passed down the windpipe and into the large airways of the lungs. The lungs can then be carefully inspected for signs of infection or tumours.
- During the procedure, samples of tissue may be taken or fluid may be injected down the tube and sucked out in order to take 'washings' from the lungs. The tissue samples and washings are then examined in the laboratory.
- After bronchoscopy, you will be asked not to eat or drink for 4–6 hours until the local anaesthetic has worn off, to prevent the risk of choking.
- If a tissue sample has been taken, you may cough up a small amount of blood over the next few days, but this is quite normal.

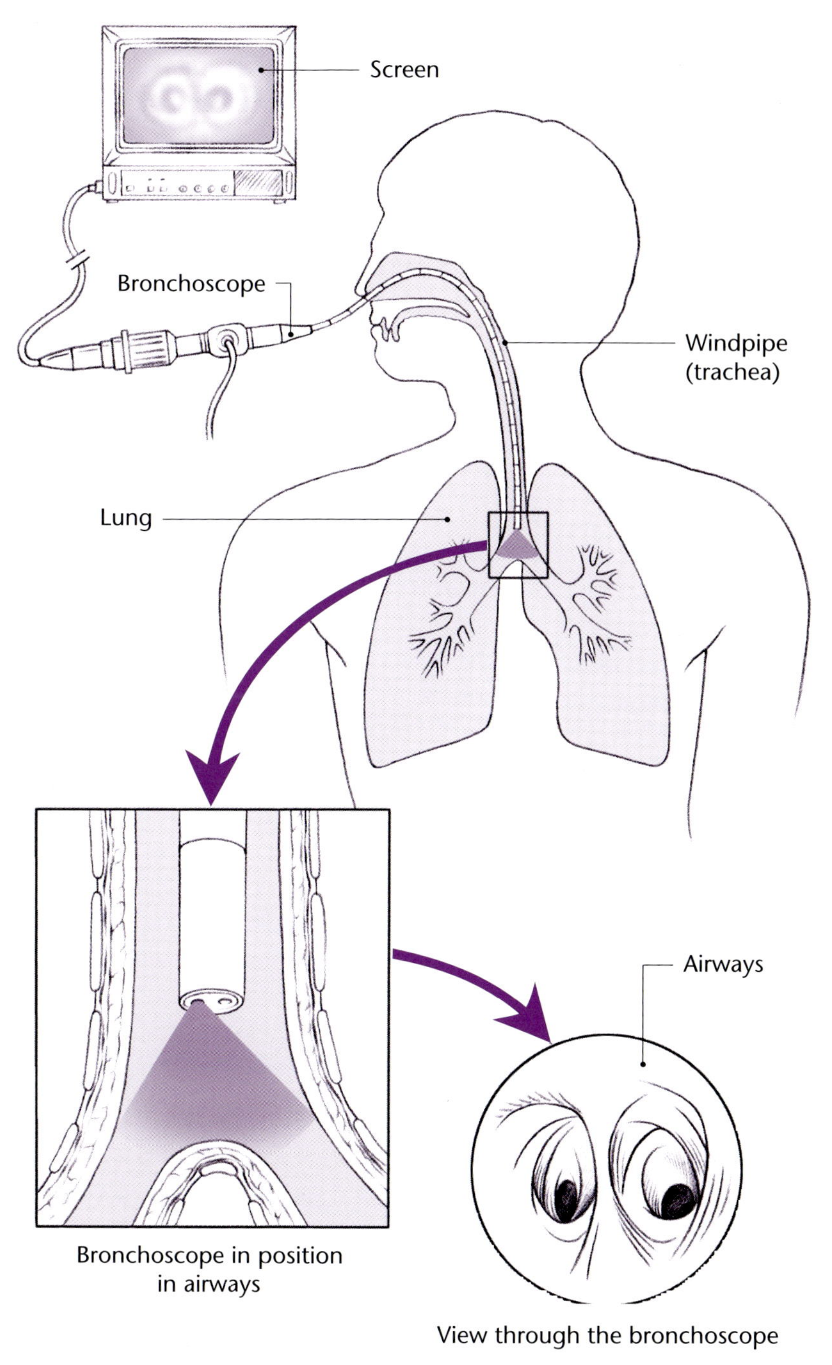

Bronchoscope in position in airways

View through the bronchoscope

Pleural effusions and pleural biopsy

- A pleural effusion is a build up of fluid in the space between the covering of the lungs and the inside of the chest wall. This area is called the pleural space. Pleural effusion can happen with pneumonia, tuberculosis, and Kaposi's sarcoma, and if you have blood clots on the lung.

- If the pleural effusion is large, it may squeeze the lung underneath it and you may feel breathless as a result. Although you may not know if you have a small effusion, it can easily be detected on a chest X-ray.

- To find out what is causing the pleural effusion, your doctor may need to take a sample of the fluid that has built up. Removing some of the fluid may also make breathing easier. At the same time as fluid is being removed, a small sample of tissue may be taken for examination. This tissue sample is called a pleural biopsy.

- It is easiest to drain the fluid from the back of the chest. You will usually be asked to sit on a chair and lean forward while this is being done.

- A local anaesthetic will be injected into your skin and a needle inserted between your ribs and into the pleural space. The fluid will then be drawn off into the syringe. A special needle may be used to take a tiny pleural biopsy at the same time. The procedure can be repeated if more fluid accumulates.

- Removal of fluid and pleural biopsy are usually out-patient procedures. You may feel a bit of discomfort afterwards, but this can be treated with painkillers.

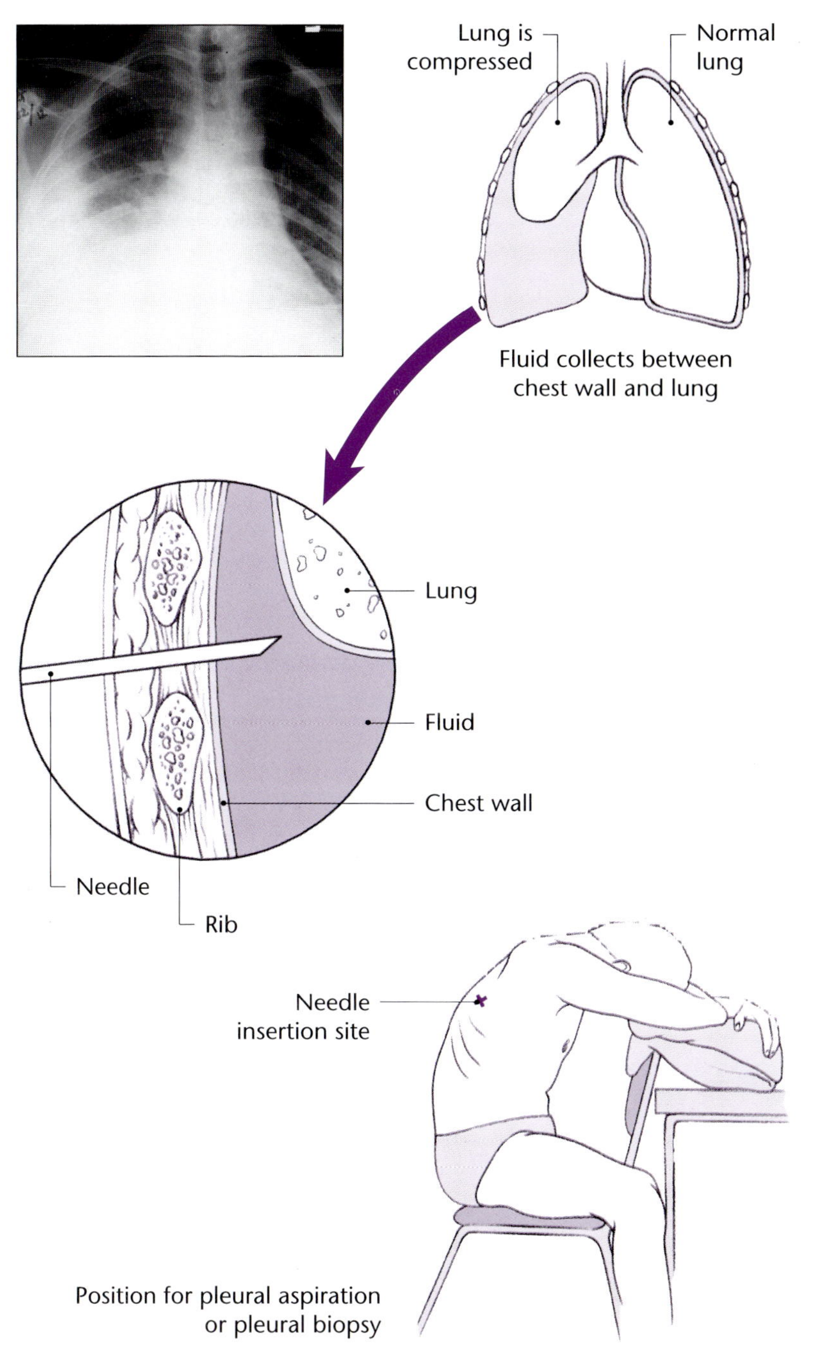
Lung is compressed
Normal lung
Fluid collects between chest wall and lung
Lung
Fluid
Chest wall
Needle
Rib
Needle insertion site
Position for pleural aspiration or pleural biopsy

Pneumothorax

- Pneumothorax is the name used when there is air between the lung and the inside of the chest, an area called the pleural space. Pneumothorax happens if the lung collapses, which usually results from a small leak developing on the lung surface.

- The most common causes of pneumothorax in people with HIV infection are lung infections such as *Pneumocystis carinii* pneumonia and tuberculosis.

- The symptoms of pneumothorax usually include shortness of breath and chest pain.

- If there is only a small amount of air in the pleural space, the pneumothorax may clear up without treatment. If there is a lot of air, however, the air must be drawn out through a tube, and this must be done in hospital.

- For this procedure, you will usually sit on a bed and you may be given a sedative to help you relax. A local anaesthetic is injected into the skin lying over the air and a drainage tube is passed into the space occupied by the air and stitched into place.

- The air passes out through the tube until the leak seals itself and the lung inflates fully. This usually takes several days and your lung will be checked on a chest X-ray before the tube is removed.

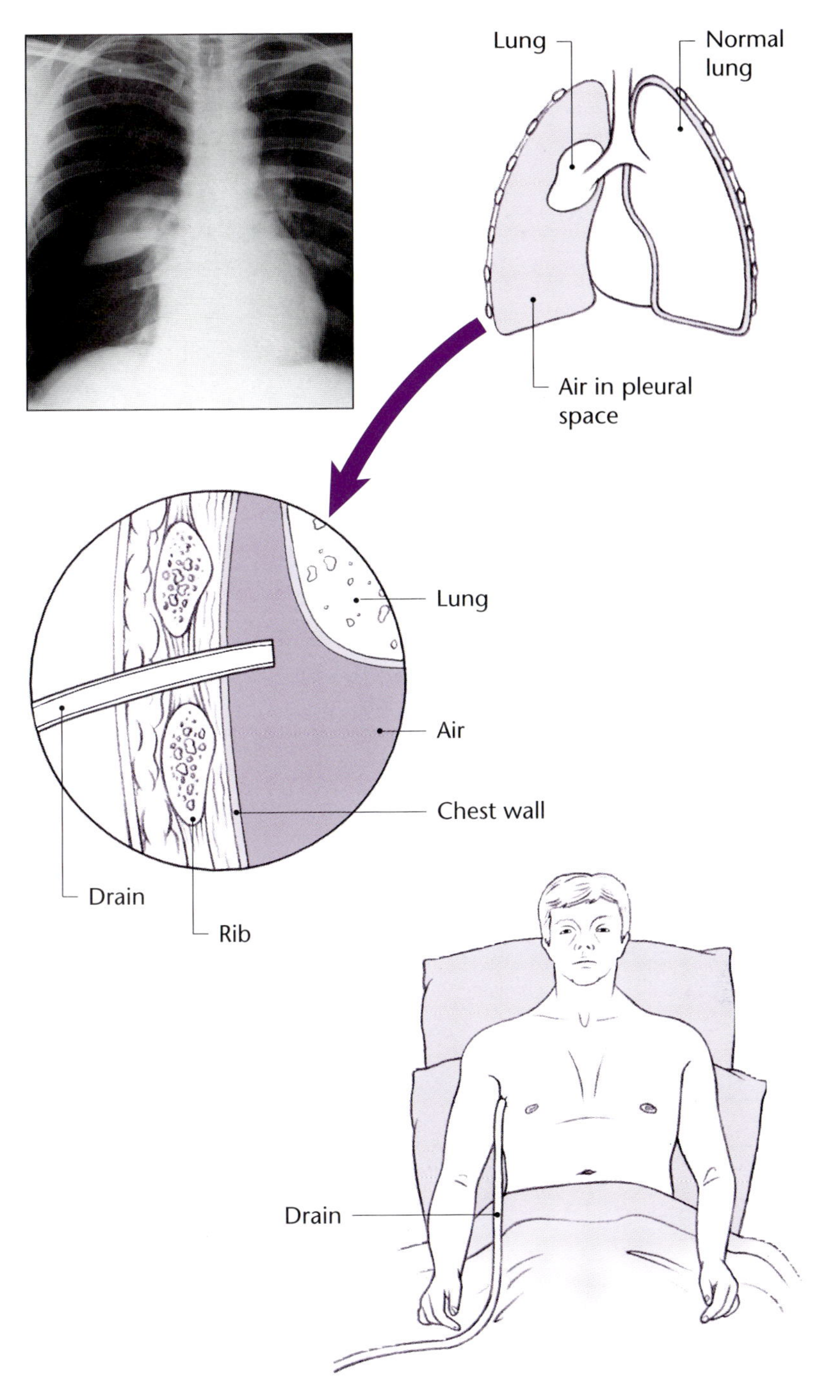
Lung
Normal lung
Air in pleural space
Lung
Air
Chest wall
Drain
Rib
Drain

Endoscopy

- With endoscopy, a flexible fibre-optic 'telescope' called an endoscope is used to examine the inside of your digestive tract.
- Endoscopy can be used to find out the cause of pain when swallowing, abdominal pain and, sometimes, the cause of diarrhoea. It may also be used to look for the tumours called Kaposi's sarcoma, which can occur inside the digestive tract.
- Endoscopy is usually carried out as a day-case procedure. You will be asked to fast overnight or for at least 6 hours beforehand to make sure that your stomach is completely empty.
- Local anaesthetic is sprayed onto the back of the throat and you are given a sedative drug. A plastic mouthguard is placed between your teeth, and the endoscope is passed down your throat, into the oesophagus and then into the stomach.
- The upper part of the gut is then carefully inspected. If abnormalities are seen, a tiny piece of tissue called a biopsy is removed for examination in the laboratory.
- At the end of the procedure, the endoscope is removed and you will be kept in the endoscopy unit until you have recovered from the effects of the sedative. This will take around 1–2 hours.
- Once the local anaesthetic has worn off (after about 1–2 hours), you will be allowed to have a drink and may be allowed home if there is someone who can go with you. You shouldn't drive for 24 hours after the procedure, because of the effects of the sedative.

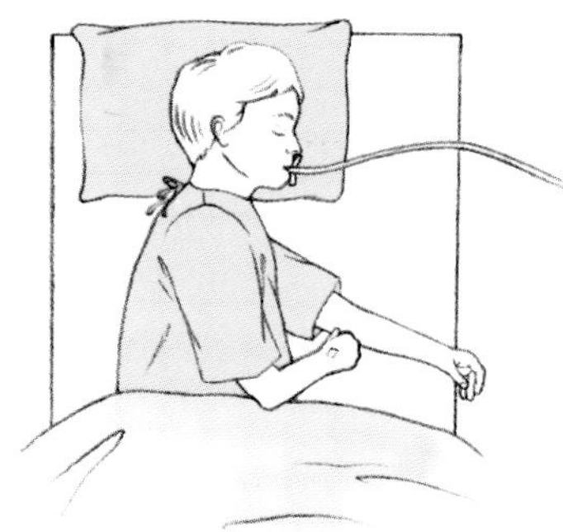

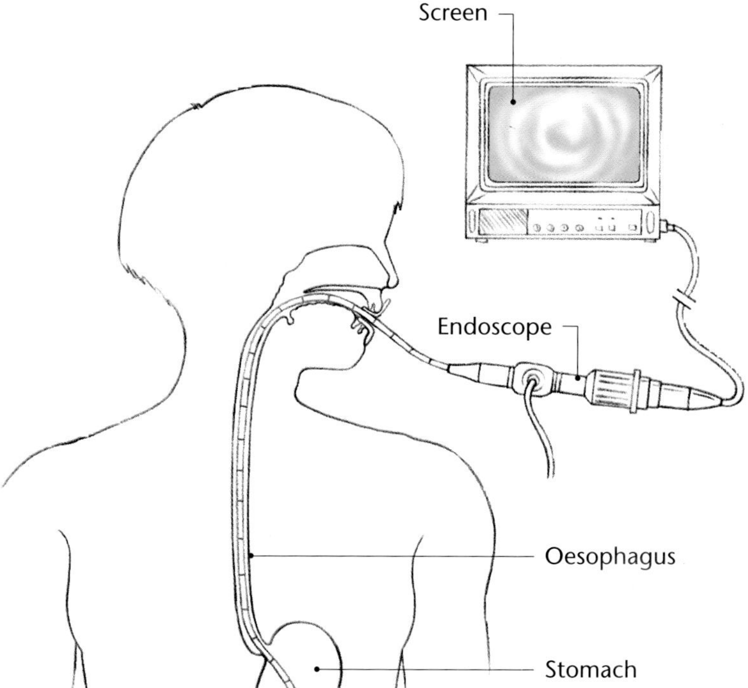

Screen

Endoscope

Oesophagus

Stomach

ERCP

- Around 1 in 20 people with advanced HIV infection develop a condition called AIDS cholangiopathy, in which scarring of the bile ducts occurs. The bile is a waste product that is made in the liver and the bile ducts carry the bile from the liver to the intestine.

- AIDS cholangiopathy often causes abdominal pain, fevers and, occasionally, jaundice. ERCP, which stands for endoscopic retrograde cholangiopancreatography, can help to diagnose this condition.

- ERCP involves using a thin flexible fibre-optic 'telescope' called an endoscope to look at the pancreas and bile ducts.

- The investigation is usually carried out as a day-case procedure. You will be asked to fast overnight or for at least 6 hours beforehand to make sure that your stomach is completely empty.

- Local anaesthetic is sprayed onto the back of the throat and you will be given a sedative drug. A plastic mouthguard is placed between the teeth, and the endoscope is passed down the throat, into the oesophagus, stomach and then into the section of the intestine called the duodenum. A smaller tube is then passed down the endoscope until it reaches the opening of the bile ducts.

- Dye is injected down the endoscope and into the bile ducts and X-rays are taken so that the pancreas and bile ducts can be seen.

- Occasionally, a small cut may be made at the bottom of the main bile duct during ERCP. This procedure is painless, and helps to drain the bile and relieve pain.

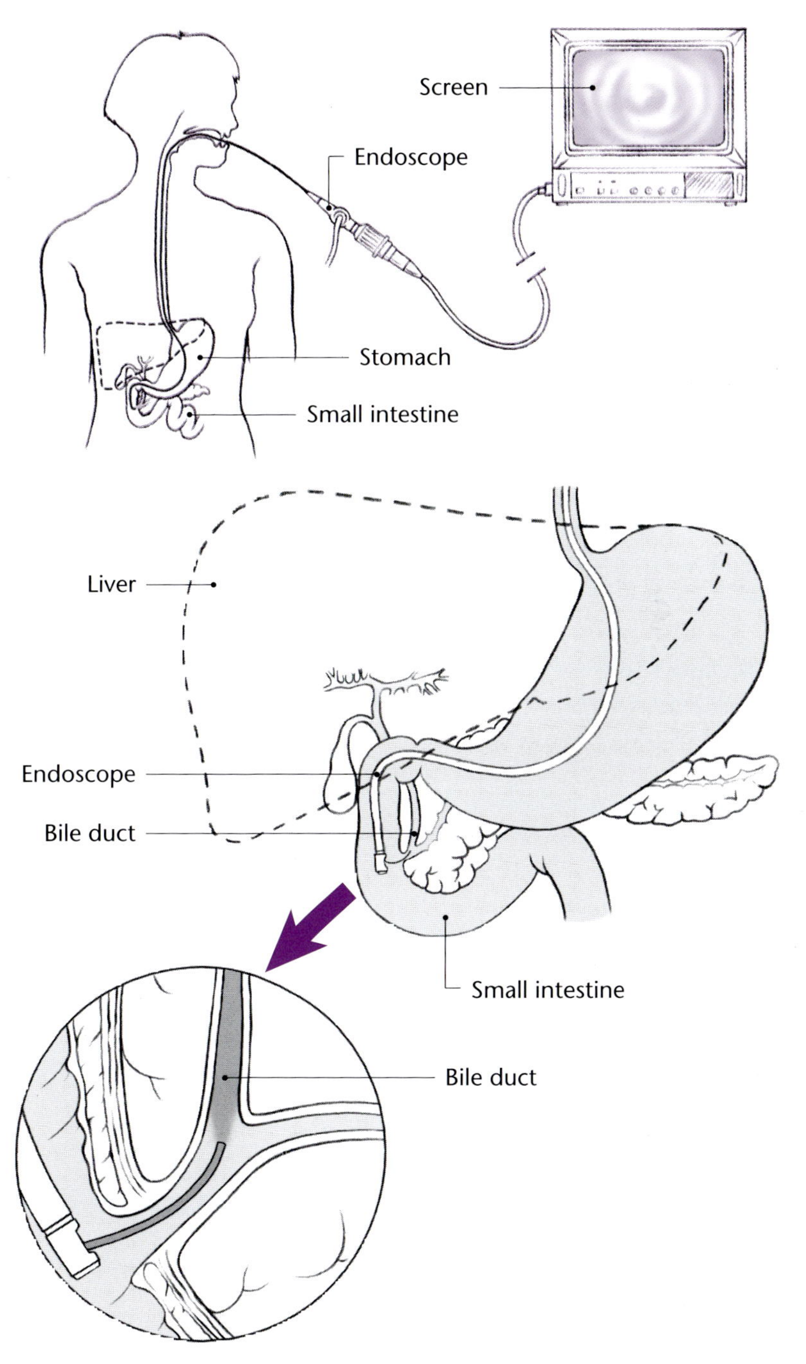
Screen
Endoscope
Stomach
Small intestine
Liver
Endoscope
Bile duct
Small intestine
Bile duct

Sigmoidoscopy

- Sigmoidoscopy uses a metal or plastic tube called a sigmoidoscope to inspect the lining of the lower part of the large intestine. It can help diagnose the cause of rectal bleeding, and can be used to investigate the cause of diarrhoea.

- During the procedure, you will be asked to lie on your side with your legs drawn up towards your chest. The sigmoidoscope is then passed into the large intestine through the back passage. Air is introduced to make the view of the intestine lining clearer. A small piece of rectal tissue, called a rectal biopsy, may be removed for examination.

- Sigmoidoscopy is painless but uncomfortable. It is the only way to diagnose some causes of diarrhoea in advanced HIV disease. The whole procedure takes about 5 minutes.

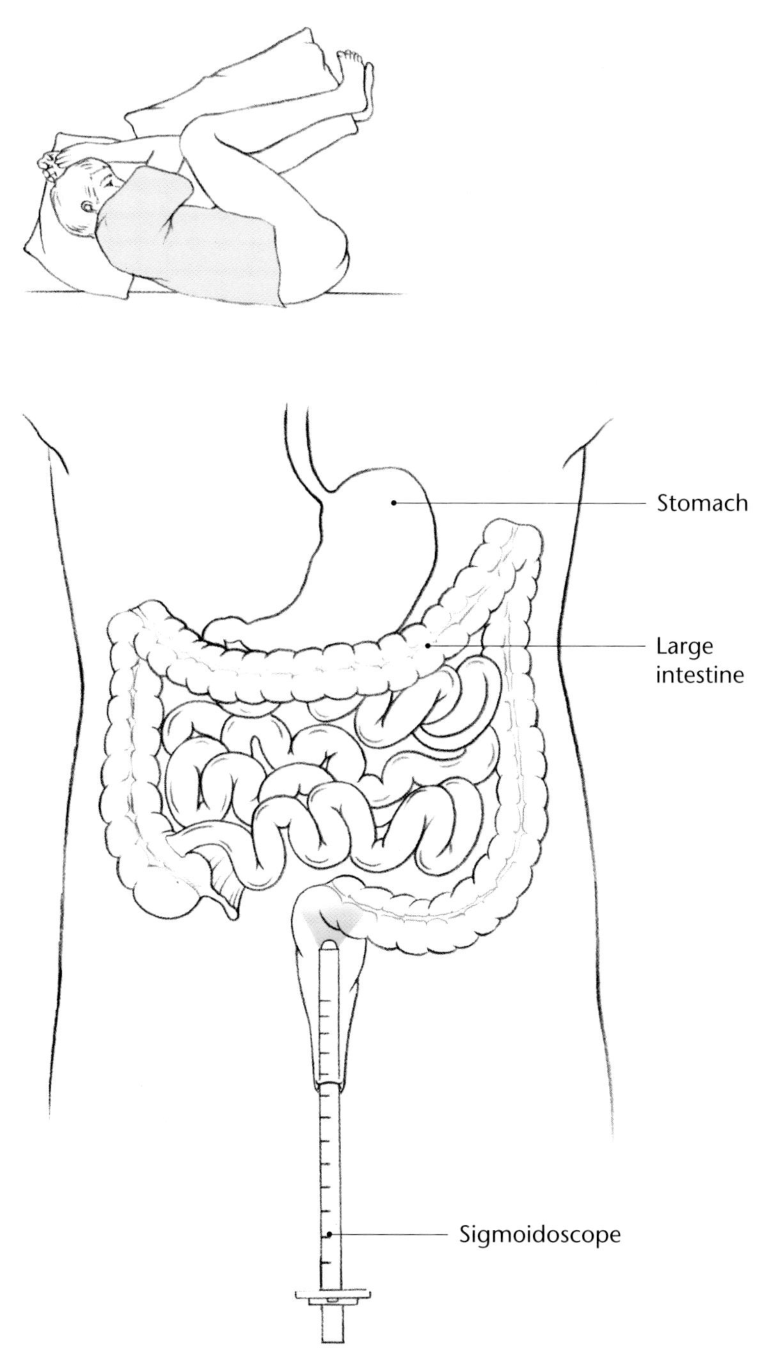
Stomach
Large
intestine
Sigmoidoscope

Colonoscopy

- Colonoscopy is a procedure in which the large intestine, which is sometimes called the colon, is examined using a flexible fibre-optic 'telescope' called a colonoscope. Colonoscopy may be carried out when sigmoidoscopy and examination of stool samples have failed to diagnose the cause of diarrhoea or bleeding from the back passage.

- You will need to take a laxative and follow a low-fibre diet for 1–2 days before your colonoscopy, to clear your bowels. You will also need to drink plenty of liquids. This is recommended even if you already have diarrhoea, but your doctor may modify his or her advice if your diarrhoea is severe.

- You will be asked to lie on a couch on your left-hand side initially, though you may be moved during the procedure. You will then be given a powerful sedative injection.

- The colonoscope is passed through the back passage and the whole of the lower part of the intestine is examined. Small pieces of the lining of the intestine, called biopsies, may be taken for examination in the laboratory. You will not feel these biopsies being taken.

- After the procedure, which takes 20–40 minutes, you will normally be allowed to go home after resting for 1–2 hours, providing that there is someone to go with you. You should not drive for 24 hours after the procedure because of the effects of the sedative.

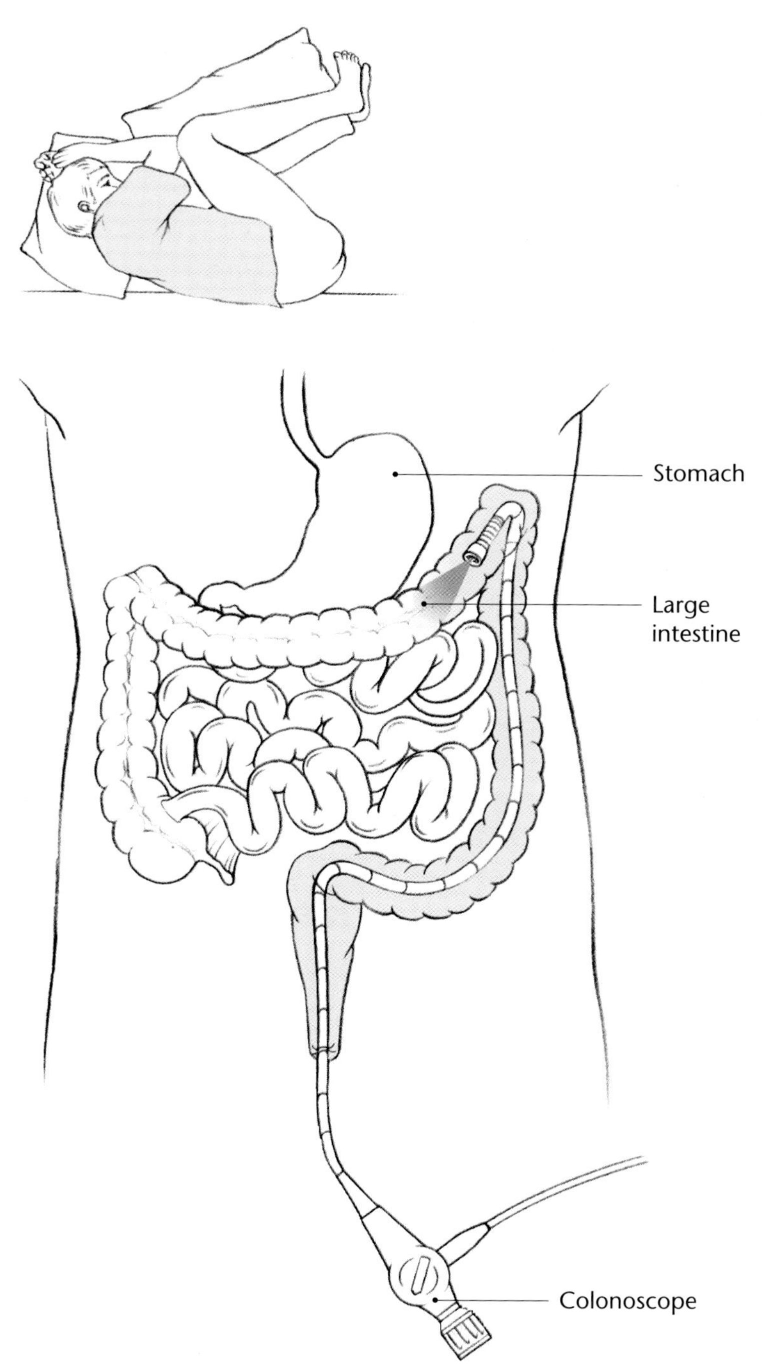
Stomach
Large
intestine
Colonoscope

Liver biopsy

- People with HIV infection may be at risk of a number of liver problems, including infections, tumours and reactions to different drugs.
- Liver abnormalities may show up in different ways, and are often detected by blood tests. However, examination of a sample of liver tissue called a liver biopsy may sometimes be the only way to diagnose the cause of an abnormality.
- Before the tissue sample is taken, a number of blood tests are done to check that your blood is clotting normally.
- Liver biopsy is usually performed under local anaesthetic and often requires an overnight stay in hospital. Occasionally, the procedure may be guided by ultrasound.
- The biopsy is taken with you lying comfortably on your back with your right arm resting under your head. A local anaesthetic is put into the skin a few minutes before the biopsy is taken.
- You will be asked to hold your breath for a few seconds while the sample is taken.
- You may feel some discomfort after the procedure, but this will be relieved with painkillers. An overnight stay in hospital is sometimes needed after the biopsy.

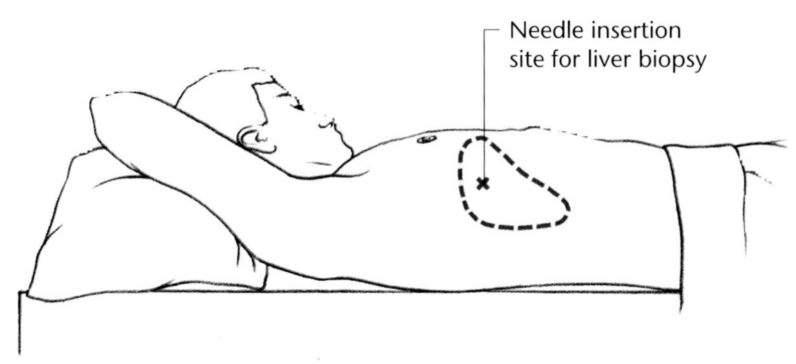
Needle insertion
site for liver biopsy

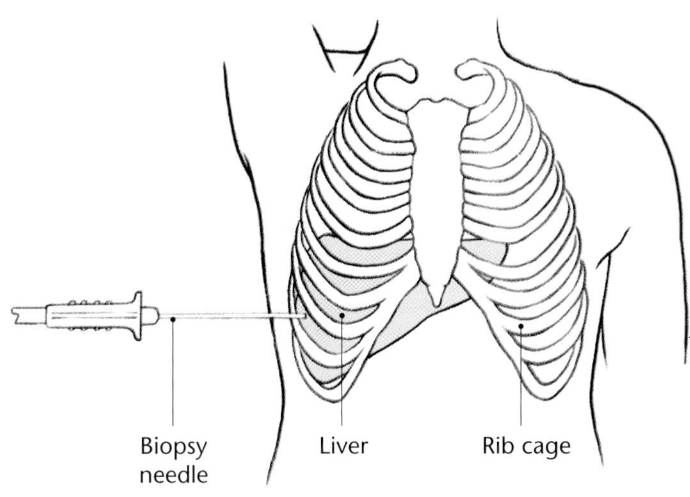
Biopsy
needle
Liver
Rib cage

Bone marrow examination

- Bone marrow is the jelly-like fluid inside the bone. It is here that most of your blood cells are made. Bone marrow examination may be necessary to diagnose some forms of anaemia and other disturbances of the blood. It can also help to diagnose some infections.

- The procedure takes only a few minutes to perform and may be carried out as an out-patient procedure.

- The bone marrow is usually taken from the right side of the pelvis. You will be asked to lie on a bed, on your left-hand side. Local anaesthetic is injected into the area from which the sample will be taken. A small cut is then made in the skin, and a special needle is inserted.

- A sample of bone marrow is taken from inside the bone, through the needle. You will feel a pushing sensation while this is being done. After this, a sample of the bone itself may be taken. This is called a trephine biopsy.

- You will probably feel some discomfort after the procedure, but this can be treated with painkillers. You can usually go home immediately if the examination is carried out as a day case.

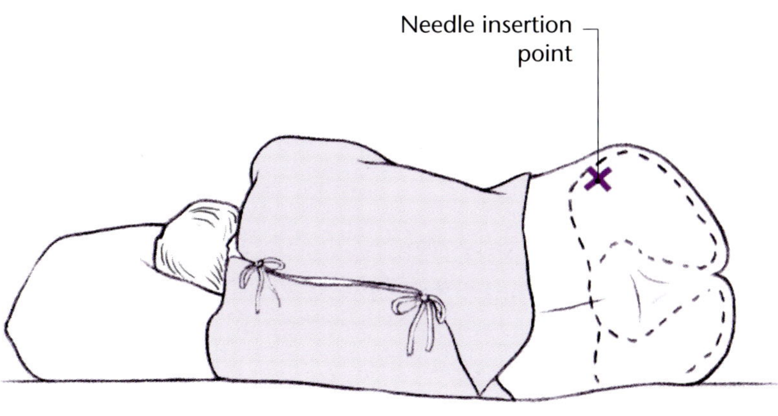
Needle insertion
point

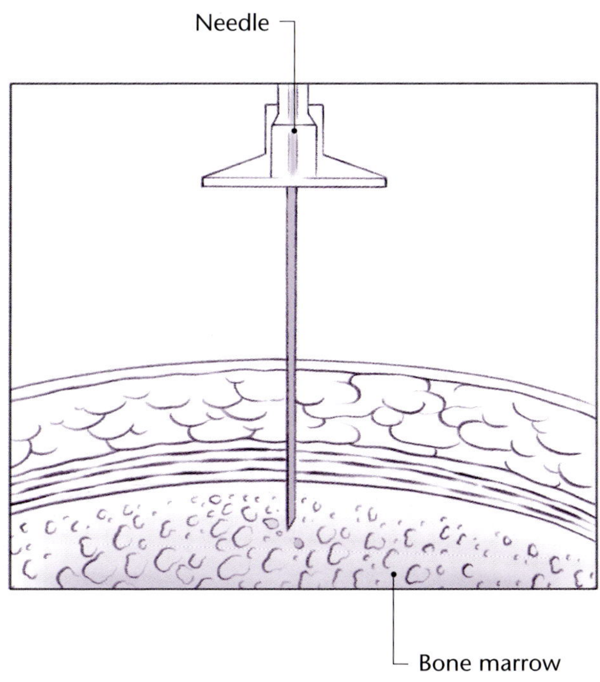
Needle
Bone marrow

CT and MRI scans

- CT stands for computed tomography and MRI stands for magnetic resonance imaging. CT and MRI scans show the internal structure of the body in some detail. They can be very helpful in diagnosing some conditions. For example, scans of the brain are often used to establish the cause of headaches in people with HIV infection.

- CT scanners use X-rays and MRI scanners use very powerful magnets to build up pictures of the body at various points, rather like slices through a loaf of bread. Both types of scanner use computers to produce the image.

- CT scanners are better at showing up some tissues, such as bone, while MRI gives the best images of the nervous system.

- Sometimes a liquid called contrast medium is injected into your blood so that the blood vessels can be seen more clearly on the CT scan. Similarly, you may be asked to swallow contrast medium so that the digestive system can be seen more clearly.

- Before an MRI scan, you will be asked whether you have any metal surgical implants. You must remove all metal objects and jewellery before entering the scanning room because metal objects may move in the magnetic fields that are produced when the scanner is turned on.

- A CT or MRI scan involves lying still for up to 30 minutes. Although some patients find being in the scanner a bit claustrophobic, it is not at all painful, though MRI scans are very noisy.

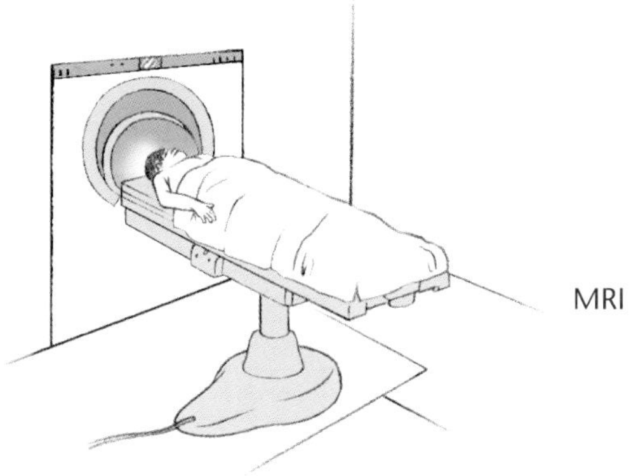
MRI

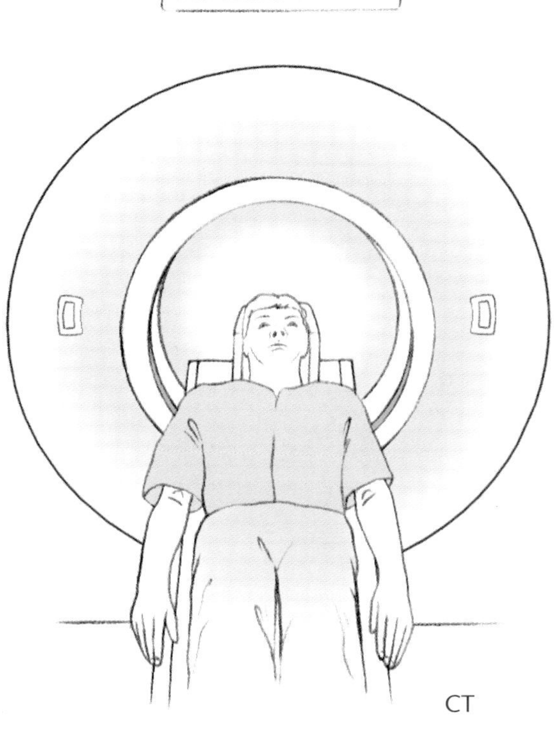
CT

Lumbar puncture

- Lumbar puncture involves taking a small sample of the fluid which bathes the brain and spinal cord, for analysis in the laboratory. This fluid is called cerebrospinal fluid or CSF for short, and can be used to diagnose the cause of meningitis and some other disorders of the nervous system that might affect people with HIV.

- Normally, a CT or MRI scan of the brain is carried out first.

- For the lumbar puncture, you will be asked to lie on your left-hand side and curl into a ball. A local anaesthetic will then be injected into your lower back. A fine needle is passed into the space around the spinal cord, and a sample of CSF is removed for analysis in the laboratory.

- After your lumbar puncture, you will be asked to lie flat on the bed for several hours. Getting up out of bed too soon after a lumbar puncture may give you a headache, but this usually goes if you lie down again. You may be advised to drink lots of water after lumbar puncture.

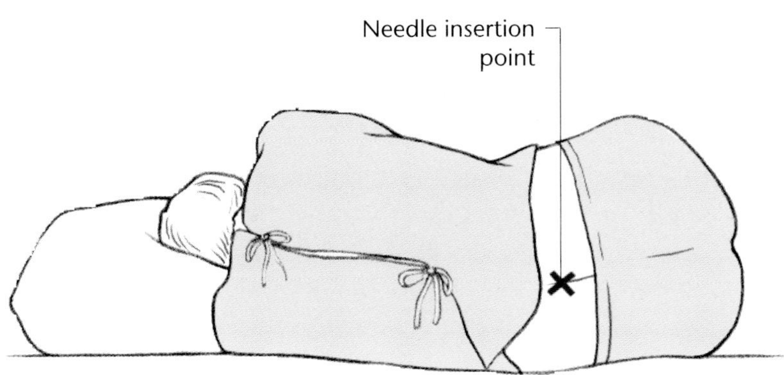
Needle insertion point

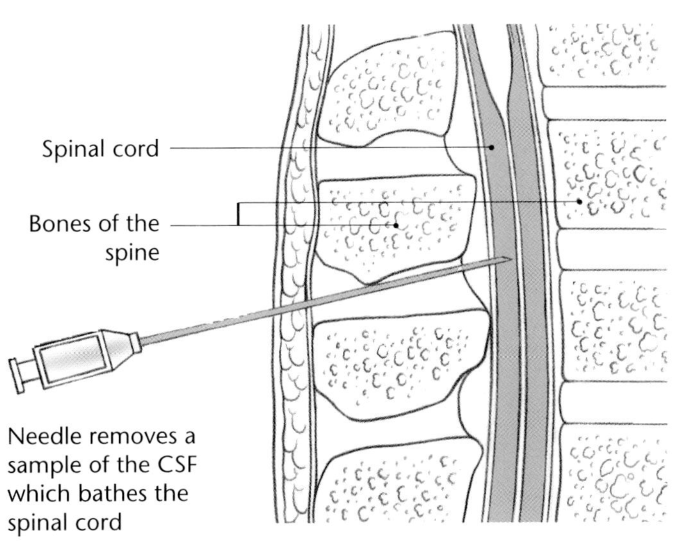
Spinal cord
Bones of the spine
Needle removes a sample of the CSF which bathes the spinal cord

CVP lines

- CVP stands for central venous pressure, and a CVP line is a thin plastic tube that is inserted into a large vein under the collar bone or in the neck. A CVP line can be used to deliver drugs into the blood, or to monitor the pressure in the heart.

- Certain drugs that need to go directly into the blood system can only be given through a CVP line because they irritate the smaller veins in the arms. Also, CVP lines can usually be left in place for longer periods (up to about 2 weeks) than can drips feeding into the forearm.

- For the line to be inserted, you will be asked to lie flat on a bed; the head of the bed will be lowered slightly. The skin of your neck or the skin just below your collar bone will be cleaned with a sterilizing solution, and the area covered with sterile drapes. A local anaesthetic will be injected into your skin and tissues over the vein.

- A needle is inserted and the CVP line is guided into the vein over the needle. The needle is then removed and the line secured to the skin with a stitch. The line is then connected to the drip or monitor, and covered with a sterile dressing. Once the line is inserted, you will be able to sit up again.

- An X-ray will be taken after the procedure to check that the line is properly positioned.

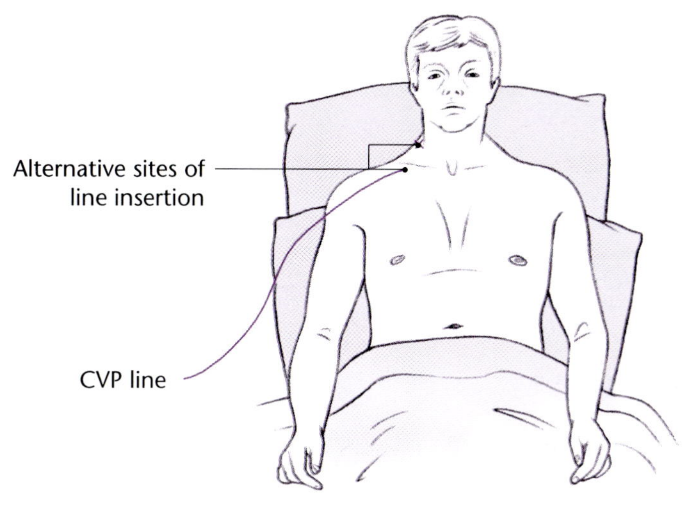
Alternative sites of
line insertion
CVP line

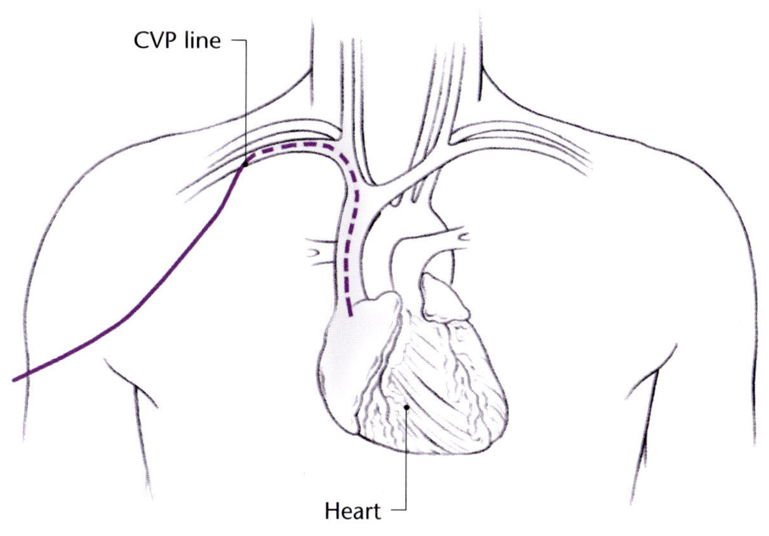
CVP line
Heart

Hickman line

- Sometimes it may be necessary to put drugs directly into the bloodstream over a long period of time, while trying to keep the risk of infection as low as possible. This can be done using a special type of intravenous line called a Hickman line.

- A Hickman line is usually inserted in an operating theatre, under either general or local anaesthetic.

- The line is a narrow tube that is tunnelled under the skin, so that the point where the line enters the skin is about 10 cm from the point at which the line will be inserted into the vein. The risk of infection with this type of line is lower because the line does not go straight through the skin and into the vein.

- After insertion, 30–50 cm of the line remains outside the chest. Once the scar has healed, it is possible to shower or bathe with the line in place, providing that it is kept very clean.

- You can be taught how to connect intravenous infusions to the Hickman line. The most important thing to remember is that you must use a strict sterile technique when giving yourself drugs through the line (see page 27).

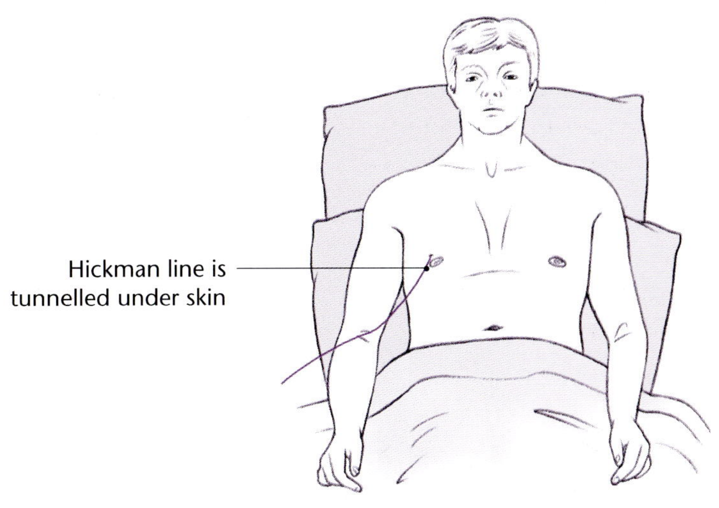
Hickman line is
tunnelled under skin

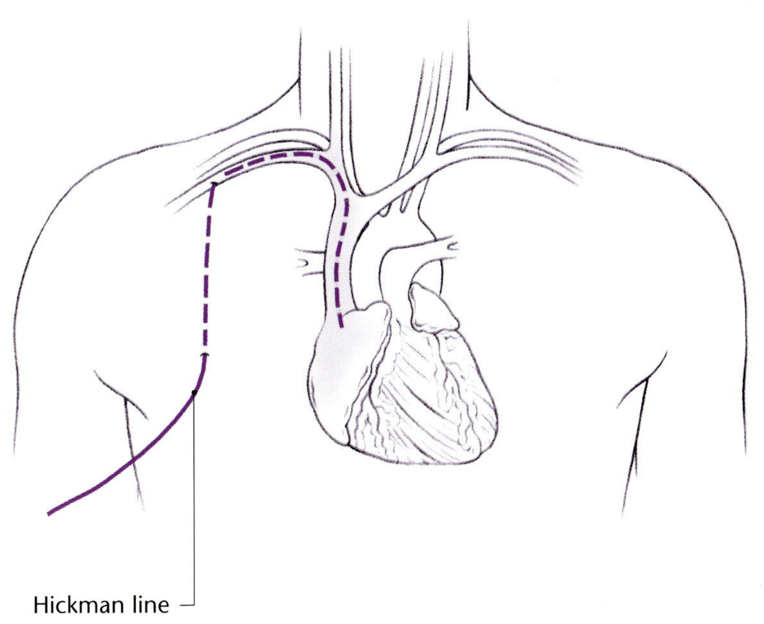
Hickman line

Port-A-Cath® and P.A.S. Port®

- Sometimes it may be necessary to put drugs into the bloodstream over a long period of time, while trying to keep the risk of infection as low as possible. This can be done using special types of intravenous line, a Port-A-Cath® or a P.A.S. Port®.

- With Port-A-Cath® and P.A.S. Port®, none of the tube protrudes out of the skin, so the risk of infection is lower. Some patients also prefer the fact that, unlike the Hickman line, the tube does not run outside the chest.

- A Port-A-Cath® is inserted in an operating theatre under a local or general anaesthetic. A P.A.S. Port® can be implanted into a vein in the arm under local anaesthetic.

- With both Port-A-Cath® and P.A.S. Port®, a narrow tube or 'line' is tunnelled under the skin and attached to a vein. A small metal device covered with a silicone membrane is implanted beneath the skin and attached to the line.

- After applying a local anaesthetic cream, a needle can be passed through the skin and into the metal device. Once the needle is in this position, blood samples can be taken directly from the vein via the line, or drugs can be delivered into the bloodstream.

- You can be taught how to administer your drugs using a Port-A-Cath® or P.A.S. Port®. The most important thing to remember is that you must use a strict sterile technique when giving yourself drugs through the line (see page 27).

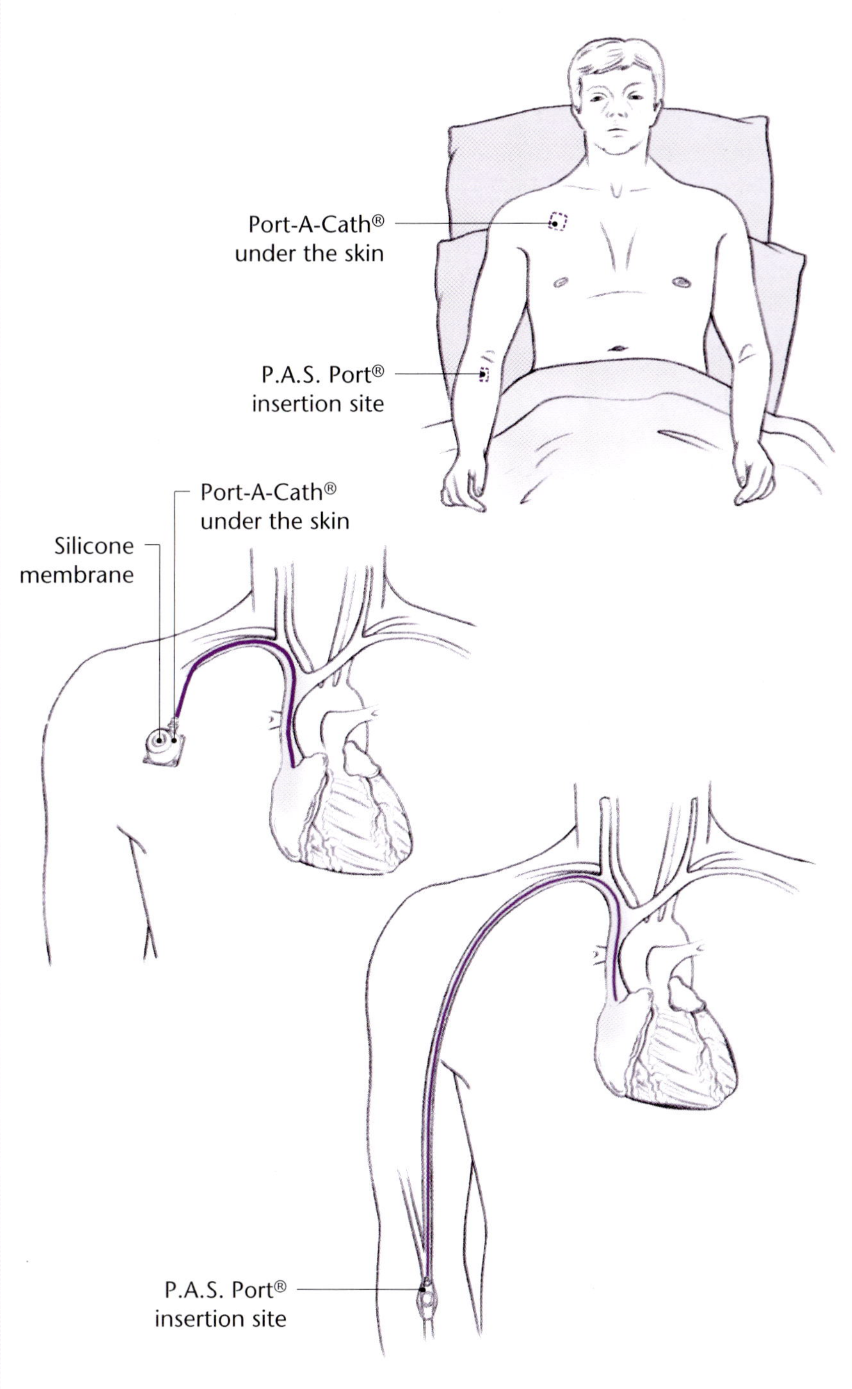
Port-A-Cath®
under the skin
P.A.S. Port®
insertion site
Port-A-Cath®
under the skin
Silicone
membrane
P.A.S. Port®
insertion site

Using and caring for intravenous lines

- If you have a Port-A-Cath® or a P.A.S. Port® you will be taught how to introduce a needle into the device.

- Anaesthetize the skin first, using a local anaesthetic cream. After about 1 hour, sterilize the skin with chlorhexidine solution. Once the skin is sterile, a needle can be passed into the metal device.

- The needles used with the Port-A-Cath® and P.A.S. Port® are specially designed so that they do not damage the silicone membrane inside the port. Ordinary needles should **not** be used. The needle can be left in place for up to 1 week if necessary, and used repeatedly while in place.

- Use a strict sterile technique when using the line. Wash your hands carefully, put on sterile gloves and get together all the equipment you will need. Sterilize the skin or the end of the Hickman line and insert the needle without touching unsterilized skin. Although tricky at first, this technique gets easier with practice and most people learn to inject their own drugs through their line within a few days.

- Hickman lines, Port-A-Caths® and P.A.S. Ports® must be properly cared for in order to keep the risk of infection as low as possible. When not in use, flush the line through with an injection of heparin–saline solution at least every 4 weeks to prevent blood clots developing and blocking the line.

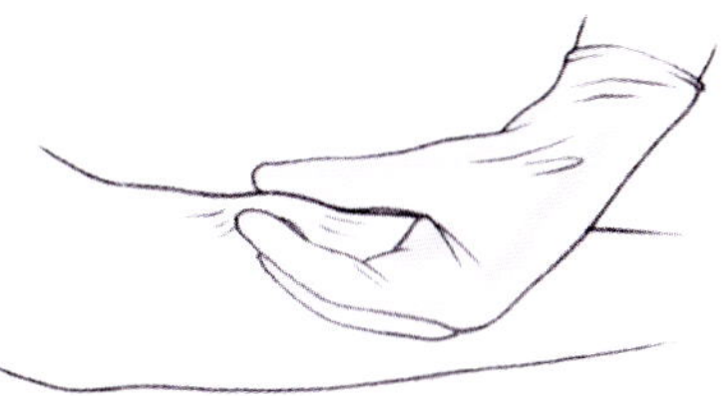

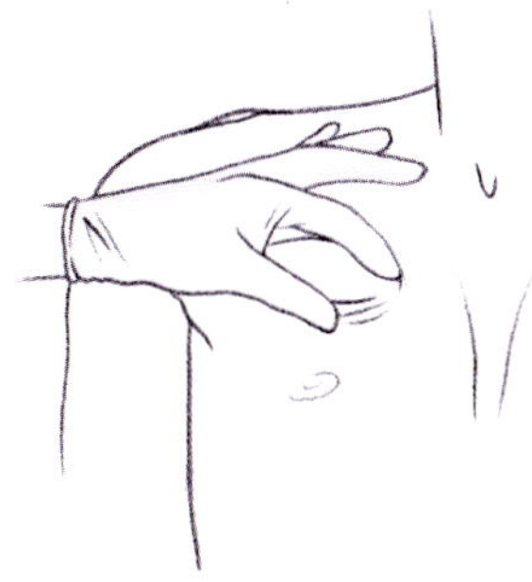

Find the metal part of the Port-A-Cath® or P.A.S. Port® under the skin

Sterilize the skin using a circular motion

Take care not to touch the sterilized skin when inserting a needle

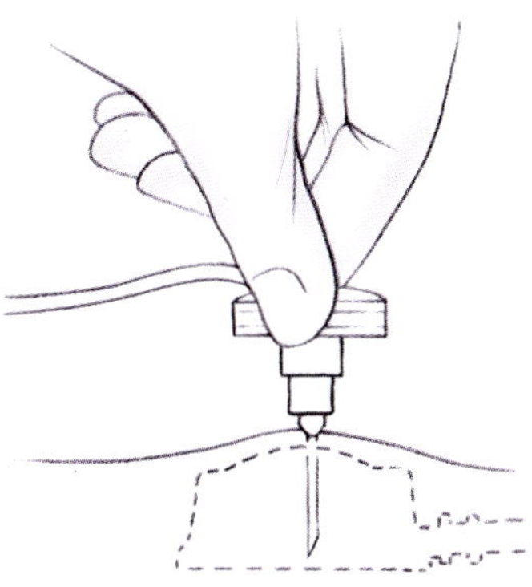

Insert the needle into the reservoir of the metal device

HIV and travel

- Diarrhoeal disease is the most common infection in travellers returning from abroad, and is the main health risk faced by travellers infected with HIV.

- New infections or fresh bouts of infections that have been previously treated are additional risks to the traveller infected with HIV. Make sure that you carry a summary of your medical history and adequate supplies of all prescribed drugs in case medical help is needed while travelling.

- Although people with HIV infection tend not to benefit from vaccinations as well as people without HIV, some vaccinations are still recommended for people with HIV who intend to travel.

- The amount of HIV in the blood, called the viral load, may increase for a short time after certain vaccinations. Because of this, viral load should be remeasured at least 2–4 weeks after vaccination.

- Some drugs used in the management of HIV disease, such as co-trimoxazole and doxycycline, may increase the risk of skin rashes after you have been out in the sun. You may also have a fresh bout of some infections, such as herpes simplex, if you spend a long time in the sun.

ADVICE FOR TRAVELLERS

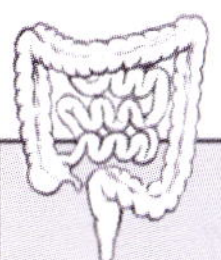

DIARRHOEAL DISEASE

- boil all drinking water
- avoid unwashed, unpeeled salads/fruits
- avoid ice in drinks

Also talk to your doctor about taking antibiotics to prevent bacterial food poisoning

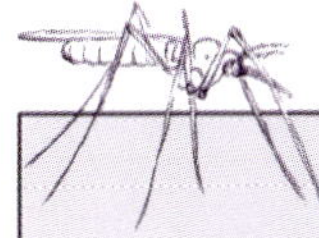

MALARIA

- avoid getting bitten by mosquitoes
  - cover limbs from dusk, when mosquitoes start biting
  - sleep under impregnated nets
  - use topical insecticides on exposed skin
  - use knockdown sprays in bedrooms
- use appropriate antimalarial prophylaxis before, during and after travel
- seek medical help immediately if you develop an illness with a fever after travelling to a malarious area (particularly within the first 3 months after returning home)

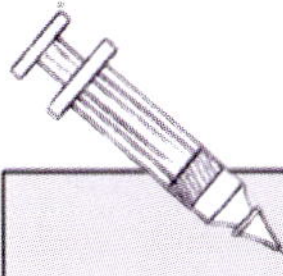

VACCINATION

Consider vaccination for:

- hepatitis A (immunoglobulin or hepatitis A vaccine, if no evidence of previous infection)
- hepatitis B
- influenza (required annually)
- pneumococcus
- tetanus

Mail Order

Additional copies of this book and other titles in the *Patient Pictures* series are available at a unit price of £10.95 (postage paid in the UK only).

Current titles include:

- Cardiology
- Fertility
- Gastroenterology
- Gynaecology
- HIV medicine
- Prostatic diseases and treatments
- Respiratory diseases
- Rheumatology
- Urological surgery

Please send your name and address, quantity required, and a cheque for the appropriate amount made payable to 'Health Press Limited' to:

Health Press Limited
Elizabeth House
Queen Street
Abingdon
Oxford OX14 3JR

Health Press titles are available at special discounts when purchased in bulk quantities for trusts, associations or institutions. Please call our Special Sales Department in Abingdon on:

Tel: 01235 523233
Fax: 01235 523238